Cultural Expressions of Evil and Wickedness: Wrath, Sex, Crime

At the Interface

Dr Robert Fisher
Series Editor

Volume 3

A volume in the *At the Interface* project
'Perspectives on Evil and Human Wickedness'

Probing the Boundaries

Cultural Expressions of Evil and Wickedness: Wrath, Sex, Crime

Edited by

Terrie Waddell

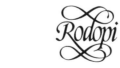

Amsterdam – New York, NY 2003

The paper on which this book is printed meets the requirements of "ISO 9706:1994, Information and documentation – Paper of documents – Requirements for performance".

ISBN: 90-420-1015-0

Contents

Welcome to *At the Interface/Probing the Boundaries*

multi-disciplinary, *ATI/PTB* publications are designed to be both exploratory examinations of particular areas and issues, and rigorous inquiries into specific subjects. Books published in the series are enabling resources which will encourage sustained and creative dialogue, and become the future resource for further inquiries and research.

Cultural Expressions of Evil and Wickedness: Wrath, Sex, Crime is a volume which belongs to the research project *Perspectives on Evil and Human Wickedness* (www.wickedness.net). This wide ranging project seeks to explore issues connected with evil, suffering, pain and the consequences of human actions. It recognises that even the language of 'evil' is a problem, and attempts to find ways of beginning to make sense of human wickedness.

Key themes that are central to the project include;

- the language of evil
- the nature and sources of evil and human wickedness
- moral intuitions about dreadful crimes
- psychopathic behaviour; is a person mad or bad?
- choice, responsibility, and diminished responsibility
- social and cultural reactions to evil and human wickedness
- the portrayal of evil and human wickedness in the media and popular culture
- suffering in literature and film
- individual acts of evil, group violence, holocaust and genocide; obligations of bystanders
- terrorism, war, ethnic cleansing
- the search for meaning and sense in evil and human wickedness
- the nature and tasks of theodicy
- religious understandings of evil and human wickedness
- postmodern approaches to evil and human wickedness
- ecocriticism, evil and suffering
- evil and the use/abuse of technology; evil in cyberspace

Dr Robert Fisher
Inter-Disciplinary.Net
www.inter-disciplinary.net

Introduction

Not much escapes the net of popular culture. I've always been excited by how the seemingly banal expressions of contemporary media effortlessly flow into and impact upon those more traditional disciplines of the Humanities and Social Sciences. Not only does the popular provide a springboard for the socially, politically and psychologically complex discourses of academic life, but it acts as a forum for intellectual debate amongst the most disparate social 'tribes.' *Cultural Expressions of Evil and Wickedness: Wrath, Sex, Crime*, was developed with this sensibility in mind. Each chapter evolved from papers presented at the '3rd Global Conference of Perspectives on Evil and Human Wickedness' held in Prague, 2002. Academics and researchers working in the UK, USA, Germany, Japan and Australia present a collection of global and interdisciplinary issues that revolve around the a-temporal and all pervasive nature of evil in the West. Some chapters touch on political, social and legally condoned cruelty, while others are more directly concerned with exploring the nature of evil in contemporary art, media and literature. Each writer forces us beyond the page. Things wicked rarely leave you sitting in neutral.

Moral and ethical transgression feed, maintain and regulate audiences, so it's not surprising that the media immerses itself in expressions of evil. Debates about monkey-see-monkey-do behaviour, inspired by violent and sexual imagery, are continually recycled by moral panics looking for a way to blame technology for 'the evil that men and women do.' As various chapters demonstrate, such behaviours existed long before the availability of modern media, as did the disavowal of social, political and personal responsibility for these extreme actions. Still … *evil* fascinates, because it has no fixed meaning – it remains a floating signifier, difficult to pin down to a definitive signified. As that which is forbidden, it is often wrapped in a sense of the exotic, the surreal, and the extraordinary. Evil makes for gripping viewing. That old news media axiom, 'if it bleeds it leads,' also extends to the larger pool of popular culture.

The material that filters through our computers, cinema, television screens, literature and music, are often post-modern fusions of narratives and ideologies appropriated from the past. That which excites and drives us, only changes in the way it is transmitted. Because contemporary visual and aural texts are often constructed with the post-modern audience in mind, audiences are necessarily be credited with a certain 'bank' of accumulated knowledge. As cultures reinvent themselves through political and religious conflict, *traces* of the apparently usurped remain to feed the collective psyche. We are products of multicultural histories and understand the popular because of our past, not despite it. Like the King Charles bridge that I walked over every day of the Prague conference, where I felt my steps echoing those that came before me and marking invisible prints for those who would come after me, popular culture connects us to a-temporal worlds.

The first part of this book, 'Wrath: purging, cleansing and appropriating the deviant *other*', sets up the connection between the past and the present. Rebecca Knuth's chapter discusses the way in which book burning, as a method of religious and political 'cleansing' by invading regimes, functions to destabilise the history, language, creativity and mythology of long established social groups. She argues that this superficial attempt to eradicate the memory and intellectual freedom of a people has been considered by democratic/humanistic cultures to be, in itself, a form of evil. As threads that connect the past to the present, books are testaments to the individual and collective contributions of bygone generations: they are, to quote Knuth, "living tissues of civilization." If the most expedient way to wipe out a people is to strip them of their mythology and language, then the destruction of books can be seen as an act of psychological genocide. From the Nazi's flattening of Poland's Talmudic Library, the burning of books in Tibet and China by Mao's Red Guards, and Serbia's bombing of Bosnian libraries, the very act of libricide acknowledges that books shape the psyche of communities. The knowledge and learning they contain, offer a sense of identity and provide the foundations through which a culture creatively and intellectually evolves. As each dictatorship crumbles, books remain. They are the defiant instruments through which communities are able to *write* and *rewrite* themselves.

When looking back on the cyclic rise and fall of cultures, it is difficult to fathom what drives a people to impose their will at the expense of others. William Cook tackles this issue, by looking at the way in which religious myths are abused by powerful church elites to gain authority and power over their laity and justify the eradication of the heathen *other*. Cook takes as his case study two specific examples - the overthrow of the Pequot Indians by the Puritans in 1637 and the annihilation of the Cathar religious sect by the Pope Innocent III and his successors. Without the powerful few to interpret 'God's Word' and so determine who should and should not be worthy of salvation, redemption and dominion over life and property, argues Cook, the Puritans and the crusaders would not have wasted entire cities of civilians. He sees the interpretation of religious myths, not the myths themselves, as potent propaganda, powerful enough to compel one race or creed to turn against another, and self-serving enough to provide a bounty of spoils for the propagandists behind these ideological distortions.

It's not difficult to equate this kind of past intolerance against those unwilling to kowtow to prescribed religious and social conventions, with the prejudice that is played out on small alternative groups today. Used as scapegoats by the mainstream for their unwillingness to conform, marginal 'cults' are frequently misunderstood and maligned. Meg Barker looks at two such groups in the UK - Goths and Pagans. Through a series of interviews with members of each group, she explores the often tense relationship between these collectives and the communities they live in. Perhaps the most recent controversy surrounding Goths and Pagans is the way in which they have been linked to violent crime, particularly the Columbine High School shooting in Denver USA, where gunmen Dylan Klebold and Eric Harris adopted a Goth-like way of dressing and presenting themselves. Barker argues, that this kind of media hype is enabled by unfounded prejudice and public ignorance of the Goth and Pagan lifestyle. Through the interviewing process, Barker discovered that Goths often link themselves to groups which have been persecuted in the past: their identification with Pagan societies, once demonised by the Christianity, echoes loudly in their discourse.

Michael Strmiska's chapter takes us back to the persecution of the ancient Pagans alluded to by the Goth movement, and the way in which history was rewritten after Christianity dominated Europe. This displacement of established Pagan cultures was, argues Strmiska, one of the most significant events in Western history. Traces of Pagan religions however, still filtered through the Christian church in the form of ancient gods who were either modified or maligned, such as the mutation of Dionysos/Pan into the devil (cited by Barker's Goths), or holy days recast as feats days. By looking at the Roman Emperor Charlemagne's crushing of the Saxons during the Medieval religious wars and the misleading histories attached to Viking culture, this chapter asks us to try and imagine a history not formed exclusively through the victor's point of view, but one that takes a more balanced approach. The ideals of tolerance and pluralism that we seek today, can be fostered by a more acute understanding of European history: "If we accept the proposition that religious intolerance is a dangerous evil that has no place in the modern world" writes Strmiska, "let us understand full well that it was just as dangerous, and just as evil, for the peoples of the past."

My study on media images of catwomen ties the previous section of work to Part II of this volume, 'Sexual Imagery: locus of pleasure, pain, censorship and reclamation.' I've always been the various ideologies that underpin the way in which women are related to the bestial in advertising, television and film. The current linking of women with cats to excite a heightened sense of mystery, suspicion, temptation and eroticism, remains a shadow of the European Middle Ages, when pagan female deities and their familiars became abject and marginal. In order to unpack some of the messages lurking beneath the contemporary female/feline morph, the historical links between women and cats are traced from the sacred nature to the subsequent 'fall' of this relationship. I argue that, we only 'get' or relate to images of catwomen as sexuality enigmatic, predatory, and duplicitous, because of the connections made between woman and cats in the past. I don't necessarily believe that advertising creatives or film-makers consciously trace these relationships, but they, like their audiences, appear to have clear reference points that shape the images they produce. The catwoman is of course not just a catwoman - she is a collection of assumptions and ideologies about the power and fear of female sexuality.

Loren Glass takes us a few steps further in the female sex stakes. As one of the highest selling and most well known American porn videos, 1972's *Deep Throat* helped put the public's desire for sexual expression on the national agenda. Despite the liberation of female sexuality depicted in the film, and many porn films of its ilk, second wave feminism of the 60s-70s used and misused this short-lived golden age of pornography in its fight for gender equality. The radical feminist extremism, which supported the Puritanism of American culture, was vehemently countered by feminist academics and those who saw pornography as a release from fundamentalism. Oddly enough it was the sex industry that helped expose the myth of a unified feminist movement. At the heart of this pro/anti porn debate was *Deep Throat's* star, Linda Lovelace, who passed away shortly after Loren Glass' piece was written. As he argues, Lovelace walked the talk that 'the private is political' by publicising how her involvement in pornography damaged her personal life. She initially felt sexually liberated through her work in porn, however in a retraction of this position, she later claimed that the industry was exploitative and had in effect shattered her sense of self. Lovelace the celebrity thus emerged as a signifier for both the 'outing' of female sexual pleasure and the 'evils' of porn. Ironically, just as women's bodies have been used to uphold and justify various religious and political inequities, Lovelace's body was used by feminists to write their version of gender equality. The imagined evils of porn and the wickedness of sexual conservatism are still publicly debated. These competing discourses of the 70s helped set in place the underlying principle of third wave feminism - that is, that no singular position can or should speak on behalf of all women.

The evil of so-called 'video nasties' along with pornography is guaranteed to send moral panics into a feeding frenzy. Censorship decisions and lobby groups that fight for the banning of these texts often rely on the old 'cause and effect' or 'hypodermic needle' model of communication to further their cause. This theory maintains that a visual or literary product has the power to directly incite certain behaviours in its audience: the extremes of violence and sexuality are often used as examples of this thinking. The fact that these theories have been rigorously dismissed by academics, media theorists and industry practitioners since the 1960s, doesn't appear to have a great deal of truck with lobbyists, censors, or the media itself (tabloid print and television in particular) who, after a particularly brutal crime, rush to find the 'video nasty' collections of the perpetrators as a quick fix solution to an extraordinarily complex series of events. It's difficult not to think of English toddler James Bulger's murder and the totally spurious link made between the video *Child's Play III* and the crime; America's Columbine high school shooting and the films *The Matrix* and *Basketball Diaries*; or Australia's Port Arthur massacre where gunman Martin Bryant's video collection became a highlight of the media reportage. It is of course much more difficult to address the intricate social and psychological roots of these events. Why tackle the too-hard issue of gun laws when you can blame Marilyn Manson or a handful of videos?

Oldridge takes Meir Zarchi's horror film *I Spit on Your Grave* as a case study through which he highlights the often inequitable decisions made by censorship officials. The film was poorly received by critics and was one of the first films to be banned under the UK's Obscene Publications Act in the early 1980s. Oldridge supports the film as a serious piece of work that tackles the minefield of gender and sexual violence. He argues that the editing decisions of the censors made upon the film's re-release, were driven by a misogynistic backlash of the very issues that Zarchi was attempting to address. Through an inspired subversion of many readily accepted film techniques, Zarchi created enormous empathy for his female protagonist who not only avenges her brutal gang rape, but doesn't get caught. According to Oldridge it was because of this narrative decision, and the fact that the male characters are placed in positions of terror by a woman who can be seen to castrate them literally and symbolically, that the male critics and censors turned nasty. Upon its 2002 re-release the censors cut the most traumatic scenes of the rape where the victim's pain and suffering was shown in uncompromising detail. These cuts serve to underplay the brutality of the rape and overemphasise the 'depravity' of the victim's revenge. While Zarchi worked to undermine the myth of rape as sexual and arousing, the censors worked to maintain it. Oldridge's argument is a convincing study on the portrayal of sexual violence in cinema and the ways in which it is condoned and dismissed.

As sympathetic as an audiences might be made to feel for a character, the reality of rape and its consequences can only be fully understood by those who have survived such an act. Madelaine Hron's chapter explores the art therapy of rape survivors. Hron's work is a personal, rather than strictly objective analysis of the images painted by rape victims and more classical and contemporary works of art that attempt to depict rape. She asks whether this type of violation can be accurately represented at all. While the work of established artists attempts to show rape in a non-personal and often politically bias fashion, either legitimising or condemning it, the work produced through art therapy aims not to present the actual event narratively, but symbolically so as to more genuinely reflect the feelings and thoughts attached to the trauma of the assault. The very act of self expression through art, argues Hron, facilitates the healing process. As a spectator of these images one is able to come to a more acute awareness of just how potently rape impacts on the lives of survivors and how all pervasive the deep feelings of shame, guilt and vulnerability attached to this type of crime can be.

Women's bodies and sexuality have stimulated both hatred and desire. At the time of writing this introduction, the Nigerian government had just sentenced, thirty year old Amina Lawal to death by stoning for having a child out of marriage. The sentence is to be carried out after she has weaned her baby. Emails in Lawal's support circulated throughout universities around Australia. Academics and their colleagues were asked to sign an online Amnesty petition to be presented to the Nigeria government. While this case captured my community's heart and prompted the usually more contained of us in academia to reach out so that we might have some small part in helping this woman, the vast majority of cases that result in the death sentence are hidden from our view, especially for those of us who live in countries where the death penalty has been abolished. Earl Martin's chapter, which opens the third part of the book, 'Crime: versions of guilt, shame and redemption,' looks not at the evil crimes of prisoners nor the suffering of their victims, but concentrates on the futility and morally irresponsible sanctioning of capital punishment. Although it has been well documented that executions don't decrease crime, the notion of 'deterrence' is still used as a defence for this sentence. Martin thus characterises legal executions as, "the unjustified killing of another" and ultimately identifies them as an evil acts. He seeks to understand why the American public and the legal system so enthusiastically support capital punishment, even though it is often seen as an "evil practice". To try and come to some understanding of this very complex issue, Martin looks at how the public is protected from the brutality of state sponsored 'eye for an eye' killing. This is done quite effectively, he argues, through the diluting effect that religion, medical counsel, lengthy legal proceedings and bureaucratization play in the process of legalised murder.

Like the mystery and red tape that acts as to hide the cruel reality of capital punishment in America, Diana Medlicott argues that that public is similarly sheltered from the harsh dehumanising of inmates that sits at the core of both 'reform' and punishment in the UK prison system. As in state sanctioned execution, prison has not proven to be an adequate deterrence for crime nor a site of rehabilitation. Medlicott therefore argues, from a British perspective, that it is extremely problematic to justify the existence of the prison system as it currently operates. She therefore asks if an ethical prison is possible. As an example of the retributive nature of prisons, Medlicott focuses her study on the technique of the unreciprocated gaze that prisons since the 18th century have adopted as a means to depersonalise. This form of punishment operates via various building structures and codes of behaviour that allow jailers to scrutinise inmates, while denying prisoners the same power: "you are the objects of my gaze" says Medlicott of this tactic, "but you are no longer the subject who can return look for look: you cannot look back at me." These contrived systems of looking, screening and hiding prisoners from public view, work to maintain the discipline strategy of prisons. Because this process aims to degrade, inmates often come to understand themselves as debased objects unworthy of agency. Medlicott sees an ethical prison as one that embraces a sense of community: where personal responsibility and autonomy are taught, maintained and nurtured in order for prisoners to readjust to civic life. The right to 'look back' is of course intrinsic to this of type of reform.

The next chapter shifts us from the stark reality of the prison system, to the fictionalised criminal. Fiona Peters unpacks this more palatable version of wickedness in her analysis of writer Patricia Highsmith's anti-hero Tom Ripley. As Peters states throughout her chapter, Highsmith breaks with the conventions of crime fiction in order to better explore the complex nuances of ethics, morality and evil. Whereas Kant understood the morality of human relationships to be about seeing people as ends in themselves, Ripley sees people as objects, of value only for their use; what they can or can't do for him. Like *I Spit on your Grave's* protagonist in Oldridge's chapter, Highsmith's Ripley is a murder who never gets caught and never struggles with the moral consequences of his crimes. Of course this lack of physical or psychological punishment for 'moral transgression' imposes an ethical dilemma on the reader/spectator, which, as we saw in the case of *I Spit*, contributed the film's biased censorship. Peters applies Kant's notion of 'radical evil' to Ripley's acts, his ambiguous relationships with other characters, his pleasure of objects, his lack of conscience, and the sense of anxiety that permeates the Ripley novels. Kant in his theory of radical evil, proposes that good and wickedness co-exists in each person. Evil is therefore not based on sin but is, according to Peters reading of Kant, "integral to human freedom, thus he shifts the debate into the arena of morality by asking why, given the fact of freedom, man might *choose* evil." This is an apt lens through which to examine the seemingly flat yet highly complicated character of Tom Ripley. Peters analysis not only takes us deeper into the idea of radical evil via Highsmith's imagination, but through her study, she allows us to reflect on our own motivations, relationships and moral convictions.

In the final chapter, Paul Davies also tackles fictionalised versions of the criminal mind by looking at the work of director Abel Ferrara. Like director Meir Zarchi's *I Spit*, Ferrara's horror/crime films were initially put in the 'video nasty' basket by censors and reviewers. Through his concentration on religious themes and issues of sin and redemption however, Ferrara's films can be read as much more than 'slasher-cum-porn' sensationalism: they are, claims Davies, a collection of narratives that pit the evil of inner city crime against those who find themselves ensnared by it. The desire for violence and revenge that distinguishes many of Ferrara's central protagonists, provides the backdrop for, as Davies argues, "a voyage of self-discovery before resolving itself in the discovery of some sort of inner, often spiritual truth." Ferrara doesn't let his characters off lightly though. Redemption is fraught with physical and psychological torment. Unlike the more emotionally 'teflon' Ripley, these fictive killers struggle with, and suffer through, the moral consequences of their actions.

As well as helping us understand how the past fuses with contemporary thought, many of these chapters ask us to view the popular media in a new light. The more that we respect the pleasure and intellectual rigour that various media, art and literary forms offer audiences, the more we will be able to melt the prejudice that exists between those who savour the popular and those who sit in judgement of this kind of consumption. I am glad that my colleagues and students at La Trobe University share this view - they may not have been so generous with their time and advice in the process of editing and writing for this book if they had not understood my enthusiasm for the project. Finally, I would like to thank the Series Editor Rob Fisher for his support and extend my deep feelings of appreciation to each contributor for their generosity, patience and commitment.

Terrie Waddell, Melbourne, Australia

Part I

Wrath: Purging, Cleansing and Appropriating the Deviant *Other*

Systemic Book Burning as Evil?

Rebecca Knuth

Modern book burning (an umbrella term for the intentional, usually public, destruction of texts) generates a range of emotions from the world audience: confusion, revulsion, sadness, anger and fear. Our response is influenced by the perceived seriousness of the incident, its overall social and political context, and the degree to which it results from spontaneous or purposeful action. Isolated instances of book burning, often conducted by religious groups as symbolic protests against heretical or offensive ideas, tend to be viewed as misguided and reactionary, but not as a substantive threat to either a particular society or civilization in general. On the other hand, the *widespread* destruction of books is a marker of an extremism that has gained political backing and thus has the power to change existing social and political orders. The large-scale destruction of books portends a future in which books are no longer seen as vessels for society's hopes and aspirations, links between past and future, carriers of identity, and barriers to mortality - in other words, a future in which the basic structures of order and peace have broken down. Because modern humanistic societies fear cultural regression, perpetrators of systemic book burning are viewed as barbaric vandals driven by a hatred of learning, memory, and civilization: as evil itself.

Reactions that link systemic book burning with evil are intensified because books and libraries are identified with life itself. Metaphors pervade our consciousness and there is a common perception that books constitute the living tissues of civilization.[1] Indeed, historian Barbara Tuchman has called books "humanity in print."[2] The vocabulary of those who destroy books admits to the same notion of vitality (they frequently describe their actions as purging, cleansing, and excising) as those who lament the destruction. Both sides are apt to liken piles of burning books to "funeral pyres", but with entirely different interpretations of the occasion. How personally the death-like associations are felt is strikingly evident in the reports of eyewitnesses. When asked why he was risking his life fighting the fires consuming the National Library of Bosnia, the soot-covered fire brigade chief Kenan Slinic said: "...they [the Serbs] are burning a part of me."[3] Modern taboos against destroying a people's written records are rooted in the universal notion that killing and maiming human beings, whether physically or mentally, is wrong.

Perceptions of evil as a driving force behind book burning are also linked with the effects of these actions on participants: linkage of book destruction with ideologies that negate the individual human being results not only in the victimization of those who lose and value books, but also of the perpetrators who may variously demonstrate passivity, programmed yet apathetic participation, or enthusiastic engagement in destruction. Chinese writer Ba Jin described his own experience during the Cultural Revolution:

> I myself destroyed books, magazines, letters and manuscripts which I had kept as treasures for years. ... I was really bedeviled ... I completely negated myself, literature and beauty ... I even believed that an ideal society was one where there was no culture, no knowledge, and of course no literary resources. I was in a trance.[4]

Ba Jin was "bedeviled" because his environment had been transformed by those who rationalized violence by projecting evil onto others and their material possessions: he sought refuge by deadening his emotions and effectively becoming a zombie.

Other perpetrators are physically as well as mentally distanced: they destroy efficiently through bureaucratic processes and seem oblivious to the implications of their actions. This involves a pervasive normative evil that is much harder to comprehend and explain than the evil associated with passion. Political theorist Hannah Arendt, after observing Adolph Eichmann's trial in Jerusalem, 1961, offered new insight into the process by which the sociocultural climate in Nazi Germany was transformed to suppress conscience and support violence:

> And just as the law in civilized countries assumes that the voice of conscience tells everybody 'Thou shalt not kill,' even though the man's natural desires and inclinations may at times be murderous, so the law of Hitler's land demanded that the voice of conscience tell everybody: 'Thou shalt kill,' although the organizers of the massacres knew full well that murder is against the normal desires and inclinations of most people. Evil in the Third Reich had lost the quality by which most people recognize it - the quality of temptation. Many Germans and many Nazis, probably an overwhelming majority of them, must have been tempted *not* to murder, *not* to rob, *not* to let their neighbours go off to their doom ..., and not to become accomplices in all these crimes by benefiting from them. But, God knows,

they had learned how to resist temptation.[5]

Arendt argues that, single-mindedness, lack of imagination, remoteness from reality, and a certain "banality of evil" allowed bureaucrats to "wreak more havoc than all [inherent] evil instincts taken together."[6]

The third type of perpetrator, in contrast, participates directly. The regime and its officials, using ideology as a rationale, support these active perpetrators who (sometimes emotional, sometimes violent) seem to manifest a latent inner beast that is unleashed and legitimated by those in power. In a mechanistic sense, one could say that an ideology, when practiced as state policy and with quasi-religious fervour, allows moral and ethical switches to be clicked *off*, and, in some, something altogether different to be turned *on* - the desire to act on dark destructive impulses, for example, to throw books into the fire and otherwise destroy a people. Novelists are especially effective in probing the world of those who are directly, even enthusiastically, involved in destruction. Aldous Huxley (1961) wrote about the gratuitous violence set in motion when normally latent tendencies are liberated by the influence of an obsession with evil organized by secular demoniacs such as Hitler and Stalin - men who are possessed by, and who manifest, the evil they choose to see in others.[7]

Active book burners view themselves as righteously engaged in fighting the forces of this evil and are generally blind to the toxicity attributed to them by those who are appalled at not only their actions but their *embrace* of the overall context of social brutality that is so often the by-product of extremism. Perpetrators are too busy reaping short-term psychological benefits from destroying their enemy's institutions and experiencing the vicarious satisfaction that such violence engenders.[8] Book burnings become the occasion for celebration of violence *per se* - as exemplified by the elation of German students at Nazi book burnings, the gratuitous torments wreaked on scholars during Cultural Revolution bonfires, and the drunken revelling of Serb paramilitaries as they shelled Bosnia's historic and religious sites, including libraries. The manufactured excitement, a potent combination of righteousness, fun and hostility, is heady and often expresses truly vandalistic elements including malice and aggression.[9] The violence permeating a society that is under the influence of "an organized obsession with evil" ultimately affects everyone: victims, bystanders, and perpetrators.[10]

As opposed to generalized emotional reactivity of non-perpetrator populations who automatically link systemic book burning with evil, academics approach the issue with determined, if elusive, objectivity. Modern scholars, who traditionally try to distance themselves from emotionality, become suspicious when the word 'evil' enters discussion, because it introduces subjectivity. For them, the attribution of book burning to evil impulses is a seductive but non-productive mindset. Explaining a phenomenon in terms of systems - the variables that put events in motion and governs their course - and studying its processes allows scholars a certain distance and a heightened sense of intellectual control. But it also tends to shift focus away from individual morality or agency. Some sociologists have decisively relocated the source of pathology from the individual to his environment: i.e., the individual, propelled into deviant activity though circumstances beyond his control, is not capable of moral responsibility.[11] New fields of cultural psychiatry, psychiatric anthropology, and cultural psychology were spawned to consider the possibility of cultural pathology - the possibility that group behaviour results from specific societal conditions and responses. For example, under the stresses of sociocultural violence, a group of individuals could reject previously held values, assume extremist beliefs, and become pathological. Prominent in this discussion is Robert Edgerton (1992) who argues that some "sick" societies have become seriously disordered as a result of pathogenic values and paranoid constructions of reality. [12]

These scholars seem to uncouple evil not just from individual moral accountability but from its usual linkage with inexplicability. Academics can, and do, explain sick societies in terms of extremism: extremists promote the destruction of written materials as goal-oriented, a function of social and political problem-solving, and the carefully justified product of struggles between competing worldviews.[13] Book burning is one of the structural components of the homogenization of discourse under totalitarianism; participation in such activity is validated and, often, rewarded. But, irreconcilably, such formulations beg the question of *where* evil (in the pathological sense) comes into play when decision-making is distorted by radical beliefs and the commission of cultural as well as physical atrocities is rationalized by extremist leaders. It raises these questions: if the study of systemic book burning provides an opportunity for confronting and struggling with the human capacity for extreme evil, is the more compelling line of inquiry the society and its processes *or* the individual's autonomy and will toward destruction? If a society, as opposed to its members, is sick, evil, and self-destructive, should the individual be absolved from accountability?

In contrast to public opinion and in line with many academics, modern secular institutions avoid concentrating on the destruction of books as evil in the traditional sense because this implies that there is no system or motivation behind it, and therefore nothing to be gained by study or analysis. Analysis, of course, by identifying the cultural stakes, highlighting the problematic nature of such destruction, and illuminating its patterns, strengthens international initiatives that seek to expand the body of laws against ethnocide and develop effective mechanisms of enforcement, such as criminal courts. As the international community assumes responsibility for the moral accountability that was once a function of religious organizations, it must base its laws and proclamations on a substantive body of knowledge, if for no other reason than that secular criminal proceedings require evidence. Setting up an international court indicates commitment to enforce laws that would otherwise be mere rhetorical flourishes and ineffectual statements of intent. With the creation of an international tribunal in the 1990s, redress for crimes against humanity became possible - redress, of course, being designed to foster awareness and the subsequent prevention of similar acts. And because trials require defendants, the international community was forced to break ranks with the structuralists and address the issue of individual accountability. There was no point in constituting the destruction of cultural objects and institutions, including books and libraries, as a crime if it was not possible to identify a prosecutable entity.

A basic underlying dilemma is whether a viable level of consensus exists as to what constitutes a crime falling within the venue of the international community, a crime against humanity. In other words, is there sufficient global recognition and condemnation of specific forms of evil and violation to form the basis for international legal measures? It appears that the values of secular humanism have been pressed into service as the basis for defining and prohibiting crimes against humanity, such as genocide, the mass murder of groups, or ethnocide, the systemized destruction of culture. What the world community is engaged in, with secular humanism providing a tenuous foundation, is essentially a cross-cultural attempt to determine universal norms and set punishments for egregious violations of these norms. The desirability of preserving cultural objects has emerged as such a norm. In a world in which books as well as works of art, whatever their individual qualities and defects, are increasingly supposed "to incorporate universal and eternal values concerning the whole of present and future mankind," their destruction has been deemed offensive to humanity and the public interest.[14]

Extremists reject these norms and, more generally, secular humanism or any value system except their own ideologically-grounded one. Indeed, ideologues are the antithesis of internationalists. As their belief system radicalizes into ideology, those in power seek to ensure conformity and transformation through control of information and ideas. When books come to be seen as capable of threatening ideological orthodoxy or policies, then book burning is adopted as a measure to eliminate challenges to the collective good (as defined by a regime) and purge alternatives. The leaders of these campaigns are rejecting the evil contemporary world and acting on the belief that only complete and radical change will produce a transformed world of political or social perfection. For extremists, each act of book burning is instrumental, a "liberating, redemptive act" for humanity.[15] They define humanity, of course, as those who embrace their programs and ideas to the exclusion of all others.

It is no wonder, then, that the systemic destruction of books is linked with mass murder. When ideological imperatives displace traditional moral and ethical commitments, the totality of commitment required of true believers, and even the passive acquiescence of the general population, leads them into a moral abyss. In the 20th century, genocide was identified as a phenomenon in which a group, defined by the perpetrators, is annihilated for usually ideological reasons. The destruction of a group's culture, referred to as ethnocide, is a related and sometimes intertwined pattern. And it has been proposed that libricide - the regime-sponsored, ideologically-driven destruction of books and libraries - is a sub-pattern within ethnocide that accounts for systemic book burnings.[16] As purposeful forms of political violence, genocide, ethnocide, and libricide occupy the same universe.

One of the most egregious examples of the modern destruction of books was the Nazis' campaign in the 1930s and 1940s against the Jews and all ideas construed as " 'un-German' [in] spirit: the rationalism, materialism, cosmopolitanism, egalitarianism, parliamentarism, pacifism, tolerance, assimilationism, ecumenism, and modernism the Nazis detested."[17] Books linked with these ideas were pulled off the shelves of public institutions, bookshops, and private libraries and consigned to bonfires. Those who stoked the fires were Nazi security personnel and students. The mood was often celebratory because the perpetrators were convinced that they were responding to a spiritual crisis by fighting decadence, corrupt Judaism (linked with intellectualism), and the effete manifestations of humanism. This spirit suffused libricidal events throughout the Reich:

> For us it was a matter of special pride to destroy the
> Talmudic Academy which has been known as the
> greatest in Poland ... We threw out of the building the
> great Talmudic Library and carted it to market. There
> we set fire to the books. The fire lasted for twenty hours.
> The Jews of Lublin were assembled around and cried
> bitterly. Their cries almost silenced us. Then we

summoned the military band, and the joyful shouts of
the soldiers silenced the sounds of the Jewish cries.[18]

Book burning and the immense social violence being perpetrated at the
same time were considered necessary steps in the creation of a fit and
purified environment for the German people. And before long, racism and
the dream of *lebensraum*, living space, for the German people led to
similar campaigns against the Polish people—six million were killed in
six years and seventy percent of the books in Poland were lost.

Mandates of intellectual or ethnic purification recurrently drive
libricidal campaigns. The Chinese Cultural Revolution (1966-1976) was,
among other things, a push to bring about a long-promised revolution by
destroying the last remnants of bourgeois reactionary thought. Bonfires
burned throughout China as the Red Guards pulled books from the shelves
of institutions and private homes and fanatically rejected traditional
culture, intellectuals, and any object that embodied alternatives to
Communism. The Red Guards, the adolescent instruments of revolution,
turned books into a burnt offering to their secular god, Mao. An estimated
one hundred million human beings suffered some kind of persecution
during the period of 1965-1975; as many as ten million may have died.
Millions of books were lost. When the Cultural Revolution was taken to
Tibet, it provided impetus to patterns of ethnocide that had begun with the
country's occupation in 1949. Tibetan culture, deeply rooted in Buddhism,
was anathema to the Communists and had to be rooted out. Under the
Communists, as many as 6,000 monasteries were turned into rubble; over
100,000 monks were imprisoned, killed, or set to physical labour; and the
majority of their texts and records were burned. The violent
implementation of Communism in Tibet, combined with colonialism,
resulted in ethnocide (accompanied by libricide) and, some would argue,
genocide.

In the 1990s, the ethnocide and libricide in post-Communist
Yugoslavia was a common feature on the nightly news, as Serbs sought
exclusive rights to contested lands within Croatia and Bosnia. Perceived
religious and ethnic differences gave impetus to racist agendas, and all
institutions of the Serbian nation (governmental, religious, educational,
intellectual) supported aggressive measures against Muslims, Croat
nationalists, and all groups who upheld the multicultural, cosmopolitan
basis of modern Bosnia. In the 'ethnic cleansing' campaigns that ensued,
Croats and Muslims were killed or driven from areas that the Serbs sought
to occupy, and all traces of their contemporary and historic presence were
expunged. Churches and mosques, as well as libraries, archives, and
museums, were levelled, leaving nothing for remnants of the targeted

groups to return to. The cost in terms of unique and irreplaceable manuscripts and archival documents, as well as contemporary informational sources, was devastating: losses included 200,000 Ottoman documents, primary source material for 500 years of history, lost in the shelling of Sarajevo's Oriental Institute, and 90 percent of the collection of Bosnia's National and University Library.[19] Predictably, a horrified global public perceived these actions as fanatical attacks on the fabric of modernity and civilization itself: opinion was shaped by television coverage and journalists on the scene, who sometimes characterized the Serbs as possessed of a kind of group psychosis.

Each of these cases illustrates the ability of ideology, whether political or religious, to override traditional taboos and rationalize physical and cultural atrocities. It is the nature of ideologies to be extreme and the totalitarian state or community serves as the ideal host or incubator for ethnocide and libricide. In pursuing the vision of their ideology, extremist leaders find it necessary to destroy all forces acting counter to that vision, be they individuals, groups, or items such as books and religious or historical texts. Diversity of thought and critical analysis is prohibited, and the state, church, media, and academic community actively endorse violent means of enforcing orthodoxy.

When Nazis and other groups embrace a culture of social brutality and deny the humanity of their targeted enemies, we are generally quick to understand their actions as evidence of evil run rampant. In his coverage of the conflicts in the former Yugoslavia, journalist Peter Maas (1996) described a spirit of evil - "the wild beast," he called it - that exists in all animals, all people, all societies; in learning of this wild beast from events in Bosnia, he wrote, we were learning about ourselves.[20] If evil is, indeed, a latent capacity within us all, then do certain compelling ideas have a unique capacity for unleashing this lurking pathology? The events of the 20th century indicate that they do. The belief that ideas could be used to better mankind and transform society, an enduring legacy of the Enlightenment, was hijacked by ideologues. As ideas became ideologies and ideologies formed the rationale for totalitarian regimes who launched aggressive campaigns to realize utopia, books became suspect. They were distractions from the serious business of transformation, threats to the strict orthodoxy demanded by the state, sources of alternative (and thus threatening) views, symbols of resistant groups, and repositories of historical facts that compromised the regimes' claims. For nationalists, books sustained despised groups and supported their claims to cultural vitality, land, or sovereignty. For Communists and other revolutionaries, books were reactionary: they sustained traditional identities and the bourgeoisie, imperialists, and dissident forces that were inimical to revolution and transformation. Extremists are exclusionary and absolutist: they are compelled to identify and extinguish the enemy and control and expunge alternatives. In their eyes, a book can easily be the tool of the enemy or the enemy itself. In extremists' eyes, books are always problematic - they have an innate potency and potential that belies their materiality. Their potential is problematic because of the link between books and ideas that counter extremism: democratic humanism, human rights and individualism, multiculturalism, diversity, and tolerance as a basis for world peace. Since these ideas are the driving force behind internationalism, the global community has a tremendous stake in preserving books.

The catastrophic events of the 20th century, culminating as it did with the implosion of Yugoslavia, raised awareness of the fragility of modernistic notions of the inevitability of progress and human advancement. There is a growing sense that we must be proactive and serve as stewards of elements that are deemed essential to a civilized world: the cultural patrimony of mankind, the composite of all local cultures, as well as the more commonly accepted mandates of human rights and a sustainable environment. Awareness of the vulnerability of cultural patrimony has been the by-product of those who have smashed the veneer of civilization in pursuit of exclusionist utopias; each library lost is now seen as a blow against all peoples. The international community has steadily increased its commitment to democratic humanism (the antidote to extremism) and international laws prohibit the deliberate destruction of cultural institutions in war because it is so damaging to diversity, pluralism, and a common global heritage.

We are moving from the helpless witnessing of cultural destruction as evil to objective analysis and criminalisation. Analysis helps us to understand toxic regimes and their rationales, and criminalisation offers a plan and platform for prevention. The political and legal channels created by international laws are beginning to counter the relative absolution previously given to individual perpetrators and orchestraters of destruction by those who were focussed on the sovereign state and institutional structures - an absolution that is based on the difficulty of attributing agency. The trial, by an international tribunal, of Slobodan Milosevic, the former president of Serbia, with its indictments for both ethnocide and genocide, clearly demonstrates that will exists to incorporate notions of personal accountability into international justice. It signals the direct engagement of the United Nations in promoting civilization, defined as, in one of its aspects, "a systematic withholding from individuals of certain occasions for barbarous behavior."[21] And it further signals that books, as well as other cultural objects, are being accorded some measure of protected status as venerated and precious universal icons.

Notes

1. Lakoff & Johnson, 1980, 3.
2. Tuchman, 1980, 13.
3. Riedlmayer, 2001, 274.
4. Ting, 1983, 148.
5. Arendt, 1964, 150.
6. Ibid., 288.
7. Huxley, 1961, 275.
8. Goldhagen, 1997, 144.
9. Cohen, 1973, 48.
10. Huxley, 326.
11. Taylor, 1973, 67.
12. Edgerton, 1992, 39 and 55.
13. Knuth, forthcoming.
14. Gamboni, 1997, 331.
15. Bartov, 2000, 30.
16. Knuth, forthcoming.
17. Hill, 2001, 11.
18. Shaffer, 1946, 84.
19. Riedlmayer, (2001), 273-274.
20. Maas, 1996, 273.
21. Huxley, 230.

References

Arendt, H. (1964), *Eichmann in Jerusalem: a report on the banality of evil*. Revised and enlarged edition. New York: Viking Press.

Bartov, O. (2000), *Mirrors of destruction: war, genocide, and modern identity*. Oxford: Oxford University Press.

Cohen, S. (1973), 'Property destruction: motives and meanings', in: C. Ward (ed.) *Vandalism*. London: The Architectural Press. 23-53.

Edgerton, R. B. (1992), *Sick societies: challenging the myth of primitive harmony*. New York: The Free Press.

Gamboni, D. (1997), *The destruction of art: iconoclasm and vandalism since the French Revolution*. London: Reaktion Books.

Goldhagen, D. J. (1997), *Hitler's Willing Executioners*. New York: Vintage Books.

Hill, L. E. (2001), 'The Nazi attack on 'un-German' literature, 1933-1945', in: J. Rose (ed.), *The Holocaust and the book*. Amherst: University of Massachusetts Press. 9-46

Huxley, A. (1961), *The Devils of Loudun*. London: Chatto & Windus.

Knuth, R (forthcoming), *Libricide: the regime-sponsored destruction of books and libraries in the twentieth century*. New York: Praeger.

Lakoff, G. and M. Johnson (1980), *Metaphors we live by*. Chicago: University of Chicago Press.

Maas, P. (1996), *Love thy neighbour: a story of war*. New York: Alfred A. Knopf.

Riedlmayer, A. (2001), '*Convivencia* under fire: genocide and book burning in Bosnia', in: J. Rose (ed.) *The Holocaust and the book*. Amherst: University of Massachusetts Press. 266-291.

Shaffer, K. R. (1946), 'The conquest of books', *Library journal 71*: 82-85.

Ting, L. H. (1983), 'Library services in the People's Republic of China: a historical overview.' *Library quarterly*. 54:134-160.

Taylor, L. (1973), 'The meaning of the environment', in: C. Ward (ed.) *Vandalism*. London: The Architectural Press. 54-63.

Tuchman, B. W. (1980), *The book: a lecture presented at the Library of Congress*. Washington, D.C.: Library of Congress.

The Destructive Power of Medieval Mythology:
A Revisionist View of the Extermination
of the Cathars and Pequots

William A. Cook

1.   The Revisionist's Perspective

The history of Beziers, a Medieval city in southern France, is inexorably intertwined with the Albigensian Crusades, the Inquisition, and the extermination of the Cathar religious sect by the Pope of the Roman Catholic Church, Innocent III and his successors, in collusion with their Bishops and monastic orders, especially the Cistercians and Dominicans. I have become immersed in the events that resulted in the eradication of this heretical sect by the Roman Catholic Church because it parallels so closely the events that gave rise to the extermination of the Pequot Indians by the Puritans in 1637, an event that I had been studying through the literature of the Puritan Divines as it expresses a total belief in, and commitment to, the Biblical myths present in the Old Testament. I had come to the conclusion, in this study, that the extermination directly related to their belief in myths that propelled behaviour resulting in the eradication of an entire people. The crusades against the Cathars together with the introduction of the Inquisition resulted in the elimination of another people. While it took approximately 100 years to complete the extermination, in contrast with the Puritan victory over the Pequots that took less than a year, the characteristics that gave rise to this action are decidedly similar.

It's clear to me, having studied these two catastrophes, that certain events of the past and the present can be more fully understood if we bring an awareness of the beliefs that compel behaviour, beliefs that in many cases are engendered by myths, to bear on the events. More often than not, these beliefs contain characteristics that are discernible and predictable, they can therefore, be used to help us avoid repeating destructive behaviour: behaviour that fuelled the crises in Northern Ireland, Palestine and Israel, Kosovo, Bosnia-Herzegovina, and Kashmir. They are also true of the myths that fuelled the Nazi regime, especially the Atlantis myths, and the myths that sent Japan surging into China in the 1930s.

I will propose six destructive characteristics that are inherent in myth by following a brief account of the Puritan war against the Pequots and a similar review of the events surrounding the extermination of the Cathars. But before I do that, I need to confront our historians, since a primary focus of this paper is to investigate the recording of historical events: this not only allows for a contemporary perspective to be brought to the analysis of myth, but insists on it if the historical recounting is to have any impact on the present. And should the recording have no such impact, why bother? I come to this study as a researcher in mythology, and consequently, bring with me the mythologists' concern for the function of myths. One of my concerns is pedagogical; if we do not learn the truth about historical events we are the willing victims of those who would delude us. This perspective is at odds with many write about the past. It is therefore necessary to take these other approaches into consideration.

Some will contend that it is not the historian's role to judge the past, just to present the relevant facts. As Marshall Smelser says regarding the first American explorers, "history is more concerned with the contemporaries and successors of Columbus who unveiled and populated the New World", an approach that permits Columbus to be the 'discoverer' of the 'New World', rather than taking into account the reality of those who first arrived whether Roman, Norse, or Irish for example.[1] Others will assert that it is the historian's role to present the facts with some analysis and interpretation: a position Thomas Jefferson Wertenbaker takes when he asserts that, "The task of the historian is not so much to praise or condemn as to analyze and interpret. It should be less his concern that the men with whom he deals were pious or intolerant or kind or bigoted than to explain why."[2] The result of this approach will cater, of necessity, to the reasoning provided by those being reviewed, as Wertenbaker notes: "... I have tried to be fair to the leaders of the Massachusetts Bible State by presenting their ideals, their points of view, their defense of their conduct in their own words."[3] What is left unsaid in this reporting are the 'words' of the Pequots. Other historians will categorically state their position on peoples and events thus warning us of their prejudice, although they rarely state that their opinion is bias or worse: this is the case with Samuel Elliot Morison who observed that the indigenous peoples of America were nothing more than, "pagans expecting short and brutish lives, void of hope for any future ... stone age savages ... [who] turned ferociously on Europeans who have attempted to civilize them."[4] These 'historical judgments' obviate the need to 'analyze or interpret', or question, behavioural motives. Other more recent historians take an anthropological approach to events, searching out the core beliefs that might explain those events. Jane Tomkins can be used as an example when she argues, as David Stannard notes: "racism could not have existed in early American colonial society because white people at that time were unanimous in their racist opinions...."[5] In short, if the historian can find a cultural 'norm' that explains behaviour, there should be no critique of that behaviour. Needless to say, this approach, which determines morality as it reflects the opinion of a majority of a population, removes the historian from her role as interpreter and disallows judgment whether of that peculiar institution of slavery or of the Nazi attempt to exterminate the Jews, the abnormal, or the Gypsies. And, finally, there is a group of recent historians, like Francis Jennings, David Stannard and Richard Drinnon, who venture to proclaim that it is the historian's responsibility to address the events of the past by questioning both 'how' and 'why' these events took place, and through this understanding, offer suggestions as to how they can be detected and anticipated, in order to avoid future repetition. Some call this revisionist history, implying that the imposition of today's perspective is not a valid entrance to the past. Given the historian's 'white wash' of the reality of America's past, relative to the indigenous population and the African-American slave, I contend that nothing short of this 'revisionist' approach will do.

2.   God's Extermination of the Pequots

"On May 1, 1637, the Connecticut Court, meeting at Hartford, declared war on the Pequot Indians, a Mohegan tribe living on the shore of Long Island Sound from Rhode Island west to the Thames (then called the Pequot) and Connecticut rivers."[6] Before the month was out, on May 26, a force of over 400 led by Captain John Mason and Captain John Underhill consisting of Sachem Uncas, Narragansetts, and Puritan regulars crept into the area near the mouth of the Mystic where the Pequots had their encampment.[7] They surrounded the fenced village of the tribe and at daybreak, while the Pequots were asleep, forced their way into the village, torched the dwellings, and from their encirclement, "proceeded to pick off those who sought to escape. More than 400 (by some estimates 600-700) men, women, and children were killed."[8] A month after this slaughter, Captain Israel Staughton with 120 Massachusetts men set out to pursue the remnants of the tribe and wipe them out as a warning to others. Mason tracked the main body to a swamp in Fairfield, Connecticut and killed or captured all but sixty who escaped, "An entire tribe was eliminated."[9]

What drove the Puritans to exterminate this tribe, to torch women and children, old and young alike? Alden T. Vaughn, commenting on this slaughter noted:

> It resulted in the extermination of the most powerful
> tribe in New England, it witnessed one of the most
> sanguinary battles of all Indian wars - when some 500
> Pequot men, women, and children were burned to death
> ... and it opened southern New England to rapid English

colonization.[10]

But Vaughn sees the land acquisition at best as only a partial answer. The Puritans were prodded into righteous action by the Pequot hordes, Satan's legions, and by the Puritan's frustration with Pequot retaliation attacks resulting from an earlier (General John) Endecott expedition against them.[11] Concerning this expedition Vaughn states:

> the Endecott expedition may well have represented something even more fundamental at stake here – the struggle between Puritans and Pequots for ultimate jurisdiction over the region both inhabited. The Puritans, determined to prevent Indian actions that might in any way threaten the New World Zion, had assumed throughout their government's responsibility for maintaining law and order among all inhabitants, Indian and whites.[12]

According to John Winthrop, Endecott had a,

> commission to put to death the men of Block Island, but to spare the women and children, and to bring them away, and to take possession of the island; and from thence to go to the Pequots to demand the murderers of Capt. Stone and other English, and one thousand fathom of wampom for damages, etc., and some of their children as hostages, which if they should refuse, they were to obtain it by force.[13]

Francis Jennings, whose account of the Pequot slaughter is both comprehensive and scholarly, notes that the expedition was intended to be "highly profitable." The 'soldiers' under Endecott's command were volunteers who were to, "nurish themselves on plunder."[14]

Gary Nash in his work the *Red, White & Black* claims that all the factors motivating the treatment of Native Americans in the southern colonies like Virginia, were operative in New England - English land hunger, a negative view of native culture, and intertribal Indian hostility. But he adds that in the Puritan sense of mission, the "anxiety that they might fail in what they saw as the last chance to save corrupt Western Protestantism...", could be stalled by the Indian who stood as a, "direct challenge to the 'errand into the wilderness'. The Puritans' mission was to tame and civilize their new environment and to build in it a pious commonwealth that would 'shine like a beacon' back to decadent England."[15]

If Vaughn and Nash epitomize the viewpoints of the scholars who have reviewed this period, one could conclude that the Puritans' extermination of the Pequots had many causes. The Pequots were seen as living embodiments of Satan's demons placed there to prevent the establishment of God's 'City on a hill': the Pequots therefore represented a hindrance to the 'Mission' God had given the Puritans; they terrorized the locals with retaliatory attacks following Endecott's expedition against them; prevented the expansion of English settlements in southern New England; and, finally, posed a political problem for the Puritans since they controlled a significant land area which the Puritans believed they (i.e. God) should control.

I propose that there is a more fundamental cause that wrought the slaughter of the Pequots, one that is the root of all the above 'causes', a primary cause if you will, that gives credibility to actions that would, at a distance, seem barbaric. I suggest that all the above causes are rooted in the myths that gave credence to the peculiar tenets of Puritan doctrine. The destruction of the Pequots resides in the power of these myths.

The 'principall Ende' of the Massachusetts' plantation, according to its charter was, "to wynn and incite the Natives of [the] Country, to the Knowledg and Obedience of the onlie true God and Savior of Mankinde, and the Christian Fayth."[16] Or, as the Reverend Increase Mather put it in his "Brief History of the War With the Indians in New-England," an eight page quarto manuscript of 1675 that principally covered King Philip's War of 1675:

> the 'Lord God of our Fathers hath given us for a rightful Possession' the land of 'the Heathen People amongst whom we live' and that said heathens had unaccountably acquired - but without having been injured - some 'jealousies.' That they had remained quiet so long 'must be ascribed to the wonderful Providence of God, who did (as with Jacob of old, and after that with the children of Israel) lay the fear of the English and the dread of them upon all Indians. The terror of God was upon them round about.' There could be no clearer equation: the dread of the English was the terror of God.[17]

This is the 'Mission' given to the Puritans by their 'covenant' with God: possession of the land *he* had provided for them and the responsibility to bring the heathen to *his* faith. To the extent that the Pequots represented Satan's hordes and possessed land rightfully belonging to God's chosen, they had to be disposed of by the "armed band of the Lord" as Larzer Ziff puts it.[18] It is instructive to note, and perhaps ironic, that apparently, the Puritans did nothing before 1643 to "wynn and incite" the natives to the "onlie true God", years after the extermination of the Pequots.[19]

What circumstances existed that allowed the Puritans to exercise their will on those who came as part of the Puritan cult and on the populations that lived on the land before they arrived? A variety of scholars have addressed the demographic background of New England as well as the nature of Indian culture prior to the arrival of the Puritans. Suffice to say here that the Pequot population had been drastically reduced by disease brought by Europeans: a reduction of about two-thirds just prior to the Puritan settlement. And, perhaps more tellingly, the Pequot had little inclination to adopt Christianity.[20] If their depleted numbers and the internecine tribal wars prevented the natives from mounting any significant resistance to the newcomers, the fact that they occupied the land gave incentive to the Puritans to move against them and the Pequots reason to resist: they were used and abused as the Puritans pursued their errand for God. This was made possible in part by the oligarchic authority of the Puritan Divines to impose their will on the people. According to Thomas Wertenbaker, in *The Puritan Oligarchy*:

> In the Bay Colony the Puritan leadership had a free hand in building their Zion exactly after the blue print which they were confident God had made for them. ... For a full half century they were permitted to shape their government as they chose, they could legislate against heresy and Sabbath breaking, they could force attendance at worship, they could control the press, they could make education serve the ends of religion.[21]

Wertenbaker also points out that, "It is more accurate to call it [the government in Massachusetts] an oligarchy, since it was a government of the many by the few."[22] This is an important point as we shall see, since it is the elite (those minorities in positions of power) who determine the myths for the large community. Myths derive, according to Joseph Campbell, not from the masses but from the ruling classes, the few who create the stories that become guideposts for the many. The elite perform rituals that become the means by which communities experience myth and make them part of their lives. Campbell believed it necessary to liberate religion from "tribal lien" or the religions of the world would remain, as in the Middle East and previously in Northern Ireland, the source of disdain and aggression.[23]

Puritan theologians, the elite group that masterminded the 'new Canaan', or as they termed it "doing God's errand", believed that the physical universe was the work of God, as distinct from the idea that the visible universe was God Himself. They knew that this distinction had to be maintained: after all, for the last 1,500 years, their thinking was aligned with Medieval thought, in that the transcendence of God could not be called into question. Neither mysticism or pantheism could be tolerated. "The Puritans carried to New England the historic convictions of Christian orthodoxy," states Perry Miller, "and in America found an added incentive for maintaining them intact. Puritanism was not merely a religious creed and a theology, it was also a program for society."[24] If individuals had the right to seek understanding, independent of the ministers, then the solidity of that civil and ecclesiastical order would be threatened. This was a society of laws, but laws established under the guidance, indeed the rule, of Scripture.[25] Puritanism sought an ideal of social conformity through obedience, or, if not, through mandatory compliance. This then, was a society determined by those in authority and defined by them as, in Winthrop's words, "good, just and honest."[26] The presumption of intelligence and the belief in one's own wisdom has wrought more devastation, alienated and isolated more people, and circumscribed the advancement of human progress, than all the actions undertaken by the ignorant.

It is important to recognize that the Puritans maintained this Medieval perspective because they too, would not tolerate heresy. They understood the need for authority to intervene, as the Catholic Church's Inquisition had intervened and as Henry VIII intervened to cause the burning of thirty heretics to control errant thinking.[27] But intervention also meant force, if warranted, against those not 'elected' to be saved: those destined to the torments of hell. This was Calvinism, "based on a division of the elect and the damned that ran throughout mankind."[28] This theology grew out of Augustine's reasoning that some men are born "concupiscent rational animals" and some are "grace-endowed rational animals."[29] They also understood the battle between the forces of good and evil - the presence in the world of Satan's attempt to undermine God's will - which they made evident in the extermination of the 'heathen' Pequots. "The Indians were Satan's helpers," as David Stannard says,

> they were lascivious and murderous wild men of the forest, they were bears, they were wolves, they were vermin. Allegedly having shown themselves to be

beyond conversion to Christian or to civil life - and with little British or American need for them as slaves - ... straight forward mass killing of the Indians was deemed the only thing to do.[30]

3.   Determining God's Intent

Two issues are of immense importance here. From whence did this 'authority' emanate, and what were its consequences? It's not the intention of this chapter to present the arguments that rationalize the evolution of Christian thought, though W. T. Jones' work *The Medieval Mind* provides a good path to that end, except to note that as the Roman Empire crumbled, the Catholic Church, with its doctrine of the Divinely inspired word of God as its authoritative base, took control over both the civil and spiritual lives of the people. This was in stark contrast to the first three centuries of Christian development, when that sect was considered by the general population, as nothing more than a small Jewish cult. The times however, called for a supreme authority and a belief in a life with purpose, even if that life was to be in the hereafter. Jesus' teachings, according to Jones, required "conformity to God's will" resulting in God's approval.[31] This required an understanding and interpretation of Jesus' teachings. This role was undertaken by the Roman Catholic Church and then by various Christian denominations including the Puritans.

Much of the Christian teachings grew out of the epistles and writings of St. Paul, the leader of the Gentile mission. "It may be said" according to Jones, "that he more than any other individual, was responsible for the development of Christianity, as a distinct religion ..."[32] Of particular importance to the authoritative base of Christianity is the interpretation Paul provided:

> It will be seen that Paul first made the historical Jesus into a savior god and then built up a mythical setting for this god out of the Jewish legends and stories that he and Jesus, as Jews, knew in common. How, for instance, did we come to sin and so to require the services of Christ the Savior? For answer Paul fell back on the old Jewish myth of the creation. God created Adam, the first man, free from sin. But Adam disobeyed his Maker, and we, his descendants, have inherited his sins. Just as the sin of one man (Adam) brought death and all our woe into the world, so the virtue of one man (Jesus) saves us; and just as Adam's sin was disobedience, so the virtue by which Jesus redeems the many is obedience.[33]

This became the teaching of the Roman Church and continues to this day as the teaching of Christianity.

The church as an organization undertook responsibility of determining who would and who would not be included as a member. It also prescribed the doctrines and the dogma that would bring its members to obedience in Jesus. Since Paul had in his letter to the Romans, wrote that God had "marked out" and "predestined" some for redemption, adherence to the true faith was necessary for salvation. The Puritans subscribed to this belief. Indeed, orthodoxy required adherence to Puritan doctrine: tolerance of differences was not allowed. "Persons who accept the 'right' beliefs" as Jones says, "are saved; persons who mistakenly accept the 'wrong' beliefs are damned."[34] Those who accept 'wrong' beliefs were labelled heretics and subject to punishment, ostracism, slavery or death.[35] Justice waged by those with power in protection of their own people and their own dictates, negates justice for the uncompliant and leaves them helpless before that power. The Puritans carried out this understanding of their God given authority by linking the civil government to the church. Wertenbaker makes this observation:

> In ardent sermons they warned the people that God had chosen His own from the mass of those predestined to damnation, … that the one sure guide for the state as well as for the individual was the Bible, that the civil government, while separate from the church, shall be in the hands of godly men who would give religion their hearty support and suppress error.[36]

Obviously, interpreting the Bible was to be the role of the ministry. Michael Lambert states, in referencing actions taken against heretics in the Medieval era, that, "Scripture was to be mediated … to the faithful through authorized preachers; the base text was not to be put into the hands of anyone who might misuse and misunderstand."[37] That, too, was the position of the Puritan Divines. But what then of those who had never heard of the Bible or its teachings? Can they suffer damnation regardless of guilt?:

> Yes, the Puritan preacher says, because they are men and as men in justice they deserve damnation; salvation is theirs only through divine mercy, and mercy has not been extended to them. 'They who never heard the Gospel, shall never answer for not believing in it as

> revealed or offered,' the preacher admits, because it was
> not so made known to them, but yet they shall answer
> for that habitual infidelity whereby they would have
> resisted it, and whereby they are opposite unto it.[38]

What consequences resulted from this adherence to a set of beliefs that placed the authority of God's word in the hands of an elite few? Of necessity, we focus here on the Puritan determination to exterminate a people, the Pequots. First, according to Stannard:

> there is little doubt that the dominant sixteenth-and-
> seventeenth century ecclesiastical, literary, and popular
> opinion in Spain and Britain and Europe's American
> colonies regarding the native peoples of North and
> South America was that they were a racially degraded
> and inferior lot - borderline humans as far as most
> whites were concerned.[39]

Second, the establishment of the 'new Zion' in the 'New World' offered an opportunity to link the civil government with the church's teachings where the word of God should supersede the word of 'men'. "We came hither because we would have our posterity settled under the pure and full dispensation of the gospel, defended by rulers that should be ourselves" wrote Cotton Mather.[40] Those who came with the Puritan divines were their subjects: obedient servants to the Lord God made manifest through them. What they came to understand was not only the inferior status of the natives, what we now understand as racism, but the inherent right of their company to possess the land held by them. This was understood before they left England. As Wertenbaker notes:

> John Winthrop encouraged his counterparts to leave
> England because God had given the whole earth to
> mankind ' ... why then should we stand striving here for
> places of habitation, etc., many men spending as much
> labour and cost to recover or keep sometimes an acre or
> two of land as would procure them many hundreds as
> good or better in another country ...'[41]

This was the economic reason behind the migration according to Wertenbaker.

    That reference to God giving the land to His people, comes from the Old Testament and was understood by the Puritans in exactly the same way: "For the covenant the congregations claimed direct authority from the Bible and direct precedent in the history of Israel. 'The covenant of grace is the very same now that it was under the Mosaical dispensation," stated William Brattle.[42] They saw themselves as the chosen of God, that He had made Himself manifest to them, and that He had directed them to the new world.[43] But it went further than this: "The Lord hath planted a vine, having cast out the heathen, prepared room for it and caused it to take deep root... We must ascribe all these things, as unto a grace and abundant goodness of the Lord our God, so to His owning a religious design and interest."[44] These teachings allowed for the slaughter of the Pequots. It is clear that Christian myths gave credibility to the Puritan behaviour against the Pequots. In his interview with Bill Moyers, Campbell commented on this notion of the 'Chosen' and its provision for slaughter:

> the Ten Commandments say, 'Thou shall not kill'. Then the next chapter says, 'Go into Canaan and kill everybody in it'. That is a bounded field. The myths of participation and love pertain only to the in-group, and the out-group is totally other. This is the sense of the word 'gentile' - the person is not of the same order.[45]

Stannard quotes the Puritan Captain Mason upon witnessing the plight of the Pequots:

> God was above them, who laughed at his Enemies and the Enemies of his People to Scorn, making them as a fiery Oven: Thus were the Stout Hearted spoiled, having slept their last Sleep, and none of their Men could find their Hands: Thus did the Lord judge among the Heathen, filling the place with dead Bodies.[46]

And William Bradford added this commentary:

> It was a fearful sight to see them thus frying and the streams of blood quenching the same, and horrible was the stink and scent thereof; but the victory seemed a sweet sacrifice, and they gave the praise thereof to God, who had wrought so wonderfully for them, thus to enclose their enemies in their hands and give them so speedy a victory over so proud and insulting an enemy.[47]

Cotton Mather noted that the extermination was the, "just judgment of God" who had allowed 500-700 "who had burdened" the earth to be "dismissed" from it.[48]

These Puritan Divines represent God's interpreters on earth. The men took the words of Jesus and made them in their own image. These basic Christian myths, the foundations of Puritan thought and hence behaviour, grew out of the presumed relationship between God and His creatures: humans are conceived in guilt, live amidst evil, and must find their way back to the Creator. As Campbell says, "But when nature is thought of as evil, you don't put yourself in accord with it, or try to, and hence the tension, the anxiety, the cutting down of forests, the annihilation of native people."[49] In the words of William Bradford in 1617:

> The place they had thoughts on (in coming to the new world) was some of those vast and unpeopled countries of America, which are fruitfull and fitt for habitation, being devoid of all civil inhabitants, wher ther are only salvage and brutish men, which range up and downe, little otherwise then the wild beasts of the same...[50]

Thus the belief in myth allowed for the eradication of a people and the taking of their land. It justified racism and greed, which determined the destiny of 500-700 people who did not share, or even understand, the rationale that gave purpose to the Puritan slaughter. These are the destructive consequences of adherence to myth. The unquestioned acceptance of absolute right has been the hallmark of humankind's greatest achievements as well as its most loathsome acts.

4.   The Pedagogical Function of Myth

What do the above analysis teach us? I would suggest that it is possible to identify characteristics of myths as destructive forces. It is possible to identify these forces at work in many instances throughout history: all of which result in the destruction of others. We have much to learn and gain if we apply this analysis to current conditions, especially since our Western culture still adheres to the myths that have determined the events of the past 2,000 years. I suggest that historians and teachers confront these events from a new perspective, one that does not avoid bringing contemporary values and understanding to the analysis; does not excuse behaviour on the basis that it resulted from commitment to beliefs (an approach that would justify both the Puritans, the Nazis, and America's wanton bombing of the Cambodians); does not excuse behaviour on the basis that it was within the 'norms' established by that society; and one that brings before the student the means to analyze certain events in order to ensure that these misdeeds are not repeated.

This paper is unabashedly pedagogical in nature: it encourages the study of myth as a means of understanding human behaviour. Its approach is of necessity confrontational since it finds fault with the fundamental tenets of established religions, and sees destructive power within them. Its approach is revisionist, imposing contemporary perspectives on events and peoples whose actions are understandable only when viewed from the standards current in that past time. For while events of the past can be recounted, authenticated, and analyzed in light of their contemporary social structures, philosophy, politics, and religious values, they have little worth to us if we cannot learn from them in order to prevent past errors. By approaching the study of myth as a primary cause of human behaviour, we are addressing fundamental truths that have been the foundation of social interaction. If through this analysis we can predict the conditions that may result in the unleashing of destructive forces, we are then able to work toward preventing their recurrence.

The extermination of the Pequots by the Puritans, on the surface, appears contradictory. Why would a group devoted totally to fulfilling the word of God, having formed a 'covenant' with Him, having moved from their homeland in England to Holland and thence to America to protect that covenant, enamored of traditional Christian values, accept the mandate of their ministers to eradicate a tribe of people? Even if the 'soldiers' who accompanied Endecott were mercenaries, or those regulars who went with Mason acted in accordance with military custom, the consequence of their actions had to be accepted by the Puritan people and their ministers. While some argue that opening up southern New England to English expansion would not serve those already resident in Massachusetts but those yet to come, they were not privy to the slaughter. It should now be obvious from the above analysis that something inherent in what the Puritans' believed - something inculcated in them as an absolute truth, something they could not question - allowed them to accept, and even sanction, cruelty.

Jennings, in the Appendix to his book, *The Invasion of America,* compares the process of 'chartered' conquest in Europe and America. He observes that such a conquest, "was launched ostensibly to reduce heretics or infidels to subjection to a protector or champion of an only true religion … and clerics of the appropriate orthodoxy preceded or accompanied or followed the troops."[51] While Jennings hypothesis sees the use of religion as an ostensible tool for intervention and subjection where heretics and infidels are the 'game', I believe that in instances where heretics and God's enemies are hunted and burned (as is the case in the Puritan slaughter of the Pequots and in the Papal slaughter of the Cathars), the religious belief precedes the economic advantage and must be employed if the heads of state (the elite) are to maintain their authority. To this end, they will employ the economic 'carrot' to motivate others to join their cause and share in the spoils of their efforts. Economics is, of course, fundamental, but in these instances not primary. Maintenance of control through maintenance of the myths that control the behaviour of the masses and ensure power for the elite, is primary. When absorbed in dictatorial activity, the conscious mind of the laity responds to no *other*: the consequence is an obedient servant shackled to ritual, customs, tradition, and rites.

Six characteristics brought about the destruction of the Pequots. Each of these was inherent in the base myths of the Puritan faith. I also believe that these characteristics exist for similar events recorded in our histories where actions resulted from the fulfilment of myths accepted by one society and destructive to another. The examples are too numerous to record here. We have witnessed this in the conflicts in Israel and Palestine, Bosnia-Herzegovina, and Kosovo. Our histories have recorded similar events: the Conquistador invasion of Central America; the Atlantis myths of Nazi Germany; Japan's expansion into China in the 1930s and 1940s; and in ancient times, the Hebrew extermination of the Hittites, Amorites, and Canaanites among others. In order to demonstrate the existence of these characteristics beyond the Puritan destruction of the Pequots, I will look at them in relation to the Roman Catholic Church's extermination of the 11th century Cathar Heresy. But first I will list the six characteristics identifiable in myths that have the potential to cause significant destruction.

The above analysis the Puritan extermination of the Pequots was made possible because:

1. **An elite group designed myths for purposes of determining human behaviour.** In the Puritan instance, this elite group took existing dogma and modified it, codifying in the process standards of acceptable behaviour.

2. **The myth(s) contained the seed that allowed for destructive behaviour to flower.** That is, there is inherent in the myth a call to action imposed on those who have accepted this myth as a guidebook for their lives. The dichotomy of the saved versus the damned provided the premise for action, and the imaging of the natives as Satan's minions provided the motivation.

3. **The myth is exclusionary and restrictive providing access to its rewards only to the initiate or through him.** This

characteristic allowed for degrees of punishment to those who might tamper with the accepted doctrines, or those unable to accept those doctrines.

4.   **The culture responding to the myth must be in a state of economic, political, and social ascendancy that requires action to sustain that status.** The forces that require action can be economic, for example, land acquisition or fear of the loss of existing lands; or political, for example, the opportunity to gain more power or the opposite, the fear that power already acquired is in jeopardy of erosion or loss; or social, for example, the belief that those excluded from participation in the myth must be brought into it or removed as an obstacle of its fulfilment. Each of these conditions existed in Massachusetts in 1636-37.

5.   **The nature of the myth does not distinguish between the secular and religious spheres, but rather understands an absolute commitment of life in all its actions to the governing force.** We have seen the union of church and civil authority at work in Puritan Massachusetts.

6.   **A requisite structure is designed and employed, usually hierarchical in nature, to codify, justify, and implement the behaviours called for in the myth.** That structure was manifestly evident in the Puritan community.

5.   The Cathar Holocaust and God's Will

As a means of corroborating the analysis provided regarding the primary cause for the Puritan action against the Pequots, I will now attempt to parallel another extermination of a people by a different church group who were executed between the 12th - 14th centuries. It will not be possible in this paper to present the complete history of the Catholic Church's eradication of the Cathars or the Albigensians, as they are sometimes called, because that effort took more than 150 years to accomplish and its complexity encompasses religious, political, social, and cultural differences. Consequently, a brief summary of some of the major incidents that brought about the extermination will have to suffice.

13th century France submitted to the domination of four kings: France, as we now know it, was in fact a gift of Pope Innocent III to the Kings of France. At the beginning of the 13th century, Philip Augustus held sway in Northern France and was the smallest and least rich of the kingdoms. By contrast, the King of Aragon, Peter II, controlled land far beyond the Pyrenees, as far as the Ebro, for which he paid homage to the King of France, although in practice this meant little: indeed, the Counts of these areas, Bearn, Aragnac, Bigorre, Cominges, Foix, and Roussillon, lived under Aragon's protection, as did the viscounts of Narbonne, Carcassone, and Beziers. Both the Lord of Montpellier and the Count of Toulouse depended on Aragon's protection despite the relative independence Toulouse maintained. The entire area known as Provencal, developed its own language and discarded the Flemish French of the North, creating a unique and beautiful culture crowned by the lyrics of the troubadours. Those living in Provencal were considered to be the most cultured and educated peoples of the time.[52]

This too, was a period of great inquiry into the teachings of the Roman Catholic Church, not just by the fathers of that church, who were reaching beyond the writings of Augustine: men like John Scotus Erigena, Abelard, and Aquinas, others in Bulgaria and Italy, as well as Provencal, teachers like Pop Bogomil in Bulgaria, John I. Tzimisces in Philippopolis, and Papa Nicetas in Constantinople. Various sects motivated by the corruption in the Church, preached to a population desirous of understanding the truth.[53]

The Cathars were one of many sects, variously identified as Waldensians, Bogomils, and Humiliati, that believed in some form of dualism. This was understood in various ways by practitioners, but basically took the form of two ruling principles - one good, one evil; spirit and matter; God and the Devil - originally known as Manichaeanism. The Cathars of Languedoc, the name applied to the region surrounding Toulouse, denied the incarnation of Christ because they believed matter was corrupt and the evil it housed must be shunned: Christ could not have entered the world in a human body. They likewise denied the doctrine of Atonement believing instead that salvation was reached through a series of progressive reincarnations. These beliefs grew out of their interpretation of the book of Genesis, the Bible's flood story, God's covenant with Abraham, and the destruction of Sodom and Gomorrah. These events were caused by the Devil, called God in the Old Testament. The intricacies of their teachings cannot be recounted here, however, it is clear that the Cathar beliefs are as complex and derivative as those of the Catholic Church and, in point of fact, amount to a different religion. Both rely on the stories from the Old Testament that tell of the Creation and Fall, and God's intervention in the affairs of humankind, but differ in how those stories are interpreted.[54]

Catharists found favour with the common people and their lords because their ministers, called Perfects, lived rigorous and ascetic lives in contrast to the Priests and Monks of the Church who were seen as self-serving profligates. Cathars did not use churches, preferring to speak to the people in their homes or small community gathering places. The contrast of the Cathars asceticism with the Catholic Church's land holdings, its rich raiment's, rituals, and the splendour of its houses of worship, appealed to many. Catharism became a primary threat to Catholicism's control over the people. This contrast is pertinent to our concerns here. Where power, induced by fear, is exercised through an elite who determine what people must believe if they are to attain salvation or retain favour, the maintenance of that power depends upon the controls that can be enforced on the masses. Fear compels obedience: mortal fear through torture and the threat of death; spiritual fear through excommunication and threat of damnation.

The Cathars had no such power: they had no Pope, no central place of authority, no churches, no synods, no accoutrements of power, and no commitment to their God to bring all people to their truth, or else cast the unbelievers into perdition. In short, the Cathar faith did not require its faithful to persecute others because they did not believe what the Cathars believed. They did have friends and a committed flock who walked into the flames prepared for them by the Pope's legions if they did not renounce their beliefs. Commitment to beliefs is not evil until, and unless, others are forced to commit against their will. This is the difference in the way in which the myths are interpreted by each faith.[55]

The 12th and 13th century Catholic Church proclaimed its authority in civil as well as religious matters; it demanded and enforced allegiance through the establishment of Papal Inquisitors, Synods, Legates, and armies that took up the cross against its enemies, whether heretic or infidel. It accepted its authority as direct from God, in that God speaks through it: it believed that the coming of God was immanent, and that all were to be converted to the 'one true' faith. It marshalled its power through priests, bishops, monks, and cardinals, all under the authority of the Pope, and used the power of mystery to control its faithful. God is the Creator of all things and is, therefore, omnipotent, omniscient, omnipresent, and immutable. Jesus, His Son, sacrificed Himself to save humankind from damnation, and gave to Peter, and through him to each of his successors, the keys to the kingdom of heaven. Only through the Church could salvation be attained. This required belief in, among other mysteries, the Trinity, the Atonement, the Immaculate Conception, and the Resurrection: teachings derived from interpretations of Old and New Testament myths. This then is what we call faith - the acceptance of the mysterious, cryptic, apocryphal, incomprehensible and inexpressible.

The reality of Papal authority, both religious and civil, found confirmation in the actions of Innocent III who ascended to the Papacy on January 8, 1198, and curiously, was ordained on the 21st of February and made a Bishop the following day. Innocent believed that he, 'as vicar of God', was the only universal power. He alone was answerable for the souls of kings and responsible before God and all Christians. These are the words he preached at his consecration:

> Only St. Peter was invested with the plenitude of power. See then what manner of servant this is, appointed over the household; he is indeed the vicar of Jesus Christ, the successor of Peter, the Lord's anointed ... set in the midst between God and man ... less than a God but greater than man, judge of all men and judged by none.[56]

There is no question here whose authority held sway and where truth resided. Anointed by Jesus Christ Himself Innocent had to carry out the dictates of the Church. And carry them out he did.

Prior to his ascendancy, throughout Provencal (roughly what is now Southern France), Northern Italy, and Bulgaria, particularly Bosnia, there existed the many different religious sects (noted above) offering various interpretations of the teachings of Jesus. The Cathars influence spread widely throughout this region because of corruption in the Catholic Church. Preceding Popes had not forcefully moved against these sectaries, but Innocent did.[57] Simonde de Sismondi, the chronicler of French History, writes of Innocent III:

> he menaced by turns the kings of Spain, of France, and of England; ... he affected the tone of a master with the kings of Bohemia, of Hungary, of Bulgaria, of Norway, and of Armenia; ... as if he had no other occupation, watched over, attacked, and punished, all opinions different from those of the Roman church, all independence of mind, every exercise of the faculty of thinking in the affairs of religion.[58]

Innocent believed that if he did not eradicate the heresies and put all Christendom in fear, the kingdom of God on earth would be threatened.

Innocent did not try to convert the unfaithful, he "charged his ministers to burn the leaders, to disperse the flocks, and to confiscate the property of every one who would not think as he did."[59] He excommunicated or laid under anathema the lay leaders, the Counts, the viscounts and the Barons who harboured heretics, and placed their lands under an interdict. In the first year of his reign, Innocent appointed two monks of Citeaux, Brother Guy and Brother Regnier, to search out and pursue the Cathar heresy. Regnier fell ill shortly after his appointment and Peter of Castelnau was sent to join him. They were Papal legates to the provinces of Embrun, Aix, Arles, and Narbonne. These legates, together with their followers, traversed the provinces identifying heretics, confiscating property, and sending people to the stake. In 1207 Peter excommunicated Raymond VI, Count of Toulouse, a friend of the Cathars because he refused to allow an army to march through his lands looking for heretics. Innocent reacted angrily, publishing a Bull which declared that 'the Devil' was behind Raymond's refusal to sanction the orders of the Papal legates. That same year, in November, Innocent exhorted Philip Augustus to, declare war against the heretics, the enemies of God and the Church by taking up the cross. He proffered Philip the same route to salvation given to those in the Crusades against the infidels in the Holy Land, indulgences for sins, as well as confiscation of all goods resulting from their actions. But Philip did not take up the offer, and consequently leadership of the crusade fell to Simon de Montfort, a brave, ambitious and ruthless baron from the Ile-de-France.[60] He had much to gain in terms of title, power and land, in addition to the indulgences. The power of the indulgences cannot be overestimated: the Barons believed firmly that fighting in the Holy Land guaranteed them a place in Paradise. That same guarantee was now awarded by fighting on behalf of the Church in Provencal. Thus began what we now call the Albigensian Crusade, which mustered an army of over 50,000 according to the estimate of the Abbot of Vaux Cernay.

In 1209, the crusaders, peasants, knights, and lords, marched on Beziers. The masses - mantled now in the mysteries of God's omnipotent power, radiant in the armour of the righteous and marching to the will of God's almighty ministers - were committed to the extermination of the infidels who were pitted by the Devil against the forces of truth. Entering the city, they massacred the entire population estimated at 15,000 to 30,000 souls depending on your source, 7,000 of whom had sought sanctuary in the Church of Magdalin to no avail. That church still stands as it did in the heart of the city, a massive granite edifice dedicated to the sinner saint, now a tombstone for martyrs and a monument to Innocent's reign of terror. When the Pope's legate, Arnold Amalric, abbot of Citeaux, was asked how the crusaders should determine heretic from Catholic, he replied, "Kill them all; the Lord will know well those who are his." Not a house remained standing – everyone was slain. And this was just the beginning. The extermination of the Cathars continued into the 14th century.[61]

At issue here is the primacy of the myths as they played a major role in determining the fate of the Pequots and the Cathars. If the Catholic Church of the 12th - 14th centuries had not held that it alone had ultimate authority over all human souls along with the supreme authority in civil matters to act on this, and if the Puritan divines had not assumed a similar stance as to their authority in God's chosen land, neither of these religious bodies would have had reason or license to exterminate a people. But both churches did act through the power of their leaders, the elite ministers who controlled the machinery of the denominations and the civil government. They offered to their laity, an exclusive body of adherents chosen by God and so distinct from heretics and infidels, the reward of salvation through indulgences or the fulfilment of God's Covenant. The will of the elevated few to order the death of a people, was made possible by the religious elite's ability to sway their followers to the 'inherent truths' that arose from their self-serving analysis of Biblical stories. Invariably those in power interpreted myth, literally and/or metaphorically, to advance their own ends, retain their authority, accumulate wealth, and maintain advantageous ideological positions. Without the elite's manipulation of God's word and their assertion of His direct intervention to justify their genocide, the laity would have no reason for 'taking up the cross' to slaughter innocents. Therein lies the destructive power of the Medieval interpretation of myth.

Notes

1. Smelser, 1959, 5
2. Wertenbaker 1947 viii
3. Ibid.
4. Stannard, 1992, 13.
5. Ibid. 276.
6. *Encyclopedia Americana*, 1966, 294.
7. Ibid and Ziff, 1973, 90-91.
8. Ziff, 1973, 91.
9. Ibid.
10. Vaughn, 1971, 61.
11. Ibid., 70.
12. Ibid.,70-71.
13. Winthrop, 1853a, 192-193.
14. Jennings, 1978, 210.
15. Nash, 1992, 81.
16. *Records of Massachusetts* 1. 17.
17. Jennings, 183; also note that Jennings cites the Puritans frequent reference to Psalms 2:8 and Romans 13:2 as justification of God's gift to His chosen, 83.
18. Ziff, 90.
19. Jennings, 228.

20. Ibid., 15; see also Stannard, 11.
21. Wertenbaker, vii-viii.
22. Ibid., vii- viii.
23. Campbell cited in Flowers, 1988, 58.
24. Miller, 1940, 598-599.
25. Brocchieri, 1990, 189.
26. Winthrop, 1908b, 239.
27. Page, 1947, 20-21.
28. Ziff, 27.
29. Ibid., 9; and Wertenbaker, 16-17.
30. Stannard, 247.
31. Jones, 1969, 32.
32. Ibid., 37.
33. Ibid., 41.
34. Ibid., 59.
35. Forbes, 1964, 89. For an accounting of the New Englanders enslavement of Indians: "New England had early taken the lead and throughout the colonial period held more Indians in slavery than any other colonies except South Carolina…"
36. Wertenbaker, 18.
37. Lambert, 1992, 74.
38. Ziff, 28.
39. Stannard, 278.
40. Mather, 1702, Chapter VII.
41. Wertenbaker, 35-36.
42. Ibid., 58.
43. Mather, Chapter VII.
44. *Necessity of Reformation,* Epistle Dedicatory. Cited in Wertenbaker, 75.
45. Campbell cited in Flowers, 22.
46. Stannard, 113-114.
47. Stannard, 114.
48. Mather, Chapter VII.
49. Campbell cited in Flowers, 24.
50. Forbes, 14.
51. Jennings, 333.
52. Sismondi, 1996, 1-3.
53. Hamilton, 1979, 106-109.
54. Peters, 1980, 133-135 and Hamilton, Chapter VII.
55. Moore, 1975, 99 and Wakefield, 1969, 165.
56. Cheney and Semple, 1953, x.
57. Lambert, 1998, 92.

58. Sismondi, 6.
59. Ibid.
60. Labarge, 1962, 16-19.
61. Sismondi, 17-20.

References

Brocchieri, Mariateresa Fumagalli Beonio. (1990), 'The Intellectual', in: J. Le Goff (ed). *The Medieval World*. London: Collins and Brown, 189.

C. R. Cheney and W. H. Semple (eds.) (1953), *Selected Letters of Pope Innocent III*. Nelson's Medieval Texts, London: Thomas Nelson and Sons Ltd.

Jack D. Forbes. *The Indian in America's Past*. Englewood Cliffs, N.J.: Prentice Hall.

Encyclopedia Americana (International Edition) (1966), Vol. 7.

Fletcher, R. (1997), *The Conversion of Europe*. London: Harper Collins.

Flowers, S. (ed.) (1988), *Power of Myth*. New York: Doubleday.

Hamilton, B. (1979), *Monastic Reform, Catharism and the Crusades (900-1300)*. London: Variorum Reprints.

Jennings, F. (1978), *The Invasion of America: Indians, Colonials, and the Cant of Conquest*. New York: W. W. Norton & Company.

Jones, W. T. (1969), *The Medieval Mind: A History of Western Philosophy*. New York: Harcourt Brace and World.

Labarge, M. W. and C. Chivars. (1962), *Simon de Monfort*. Bath: Portway.

Lambert, M. (1998), *The Cathars*. Oxford: Blackwell.

Lambert, M. (1992), *Medieval Heresy*. Oxford: Blackwell

Mather, I. (1675), *Brief History of the War With the Indians in New-England. From June 24, 1675 to August 12, 1676*. London: Richard Criswell.

Mather, C. (1702), *Magnalia Christi Americana; or, the Eccleistical History of New England.* Vol 2. Reprint (1967) New York: Russell & Russell. p. 558.

Miller, P. (1940), 'Jonathan Edwards to Emerson.' *New England Quarterly.* December, 589-617.

Moore, R. I. (1975), 'The Birth of Popular Heresy', in: E. Arnold (ed.). *Documents of Medieval History.* London: St. Martin's Press. 133.

Nash, Gary B. (1992), *Red White & Black: The Peoples of Early North America.* Englewood Cliffs, New Jersey: Prentice Hall.

Page, W. (1947), 'The Victoria History of the County of Essex', in: T. J. Wertenbaker, *The Puritan Oligarchy: The Founding of American Civilization.* New York: Grosset and Dunlap. 20-21.

Peters, Edward (ed.). *Heresy and Authority in Medieval Europe.* Documents in translation: University of Pennsylvania Press.

Sismondi, J. C. and L. de Simonde. (1996), *History of the Crusades Against The Albigenses in the Thirteenth Century: The Extermination of the Cathars.* L. Gazarii Libris. (trans). Trowbridge: Redwood Books.

Smelser, M. (1959), *American History at a Glance.* New York: Barnes and Noble.

Stannard, D. E. (1992), *American Holocaust: The Conquest of the New World.* New York: Oxford University Press.

Vaughn, Alden T. (1971), 'Pequots and Puritans: The Causes of the War of 1637.' in: R. L. Nichols and G. R. Adams. (eds.) *The American Indian: Past and Present.* Waltham, MA: Xerox College Publishing.

Wakefield, W. L. and A.P. Evans (1969), *Heresies of the High Middle Ages.* New York: Columbia University Press.

Wertenbaker, T. J. (1947), *The Puritan Oligarchy: The Founding of American Civilization.* New York: Grosset and Dunlap.
Winthrop. J. (1960), *The History of New England from 1630 to 1649*, J. Savage. (ed) 2nd ed. 2vols. Boston: Little, Brown and co.

Winthrop, John. (1908), *Journal.* J. K. Hosmer. (ed.) New York: C. Scribner's Sons.
Ziff, Larzer. (1973), *Puritanism in America: New Culture in a New World.* New York: The Viking Press.

Satanic Subcultures? A Discourse Analysis of the Self-Perceptions of Young Goths and Pagans

Meg Barker

In recent years, several youth subcultures have become the focus of concerns about 'evil' and 'Satanism'. This chapter considers two such groups: Pagans and Goths. Throughout this study I will use discourse analysis to explore how the young members of these groups construct their subcultures, how they feel others perceive them, and how they respond to these perceptions. This research is based on a series of interviews that I carried out with Pagans and Goths in two different parts of England: one in the North West of the country and one in the Midlands.

1.   What are Pagans and Goths?

Paganism, especially the Wiccan branch of the religion, has experienced a boom since the late 1990s. Most bookstores in the UK now have extensive sections relating to witchcraft and Pagan beliefs. Many books and 'teen witch' kits for example, are targeted at adolescents and young adults. Most of these texts, and the people I interviewed, claim that Paganism is an ancient religion suppressed by the Christian church during the European witch persecutions. Many historians would dispute this claim, arguing that modern Paganism was invented in the early 20th century. I do not however, intend to examine the validity of the historical narratives constructed by Pagans, my intention is to demonstrate that such discourses are used to support their perceptions of the relationship between Paganism and mainstream religion.

Goth emerged in the early 1980s, with the music of post-Punk UK bands like *Bauhaus* and *Siouxsie and the Banshees*. Since the 1990s both the UK and US Goth movements have grown and Goth has become recognised as a distinct subculture. The huge popularity of Marilyn Manson has thrown the spotlight onto Goth again, although some older Goths disassociate themselves from this type of 'shock rock'. The boundaries between Goth and the extremely popular 'nu-metal' culture are blurred. *Kerrang* magazine, read by Goths and those into metal and nu-metal music, has recently become the most popular music periodical in the UK. Goth is often associated with a certain appearance as well as musical tastes: generally black clothing, silver jewellery, a pale complexion and dyed hair. There is however, a great deal of variety within the subculture ranging from Victorian-style velvet outfits to spiky fetish-wear and silver 'cyber' clothing.

Both Paganism and Goth subculture cover a diverse range of

beliefs, ideas and tastes, but are linked in three clear ways: both are positioned outside mainstream culture; Pagan religions are particularly popular amongst Goths, even non-religious Goths often wear jewellery containing Pagan symbols and take an interest in 'pre-Christian' myths; and most importantly for this paper, Pagans and Goths have been represented in similar ways by mainstream culture. Both groups have been labelled as satanic, evil and dangerous by religious collectives and the news media, where their beliefs and tastes have been directly linked to violent teenage crime.

A.   Goths and Pagans in the Media

Sue Chesters noted that Goths were rarely mentioned in the media before the mid 1990s. When they were, the depictions were generally 'light-hearted'.[1] In the last few years however, the movement has acquired a darker reputation. Two crimes in particular have fuelled this moral panic: the 1996 Florida 'vampire murders' by teenage members of a 'vampire cult' and the 1999 'trench coat killings'.[2] In the latter case two teenaged boys, Dylan Klebold and Eric Harris, shot and killed thirteen people at their Denver school, Columbine High, where they and their friends had been labelled 'the trench coat mafia'. Writing in *The Sunday Times*, Andrew Smith also links the London bomber, David Copeland, to the Goth scene.[3] In a recent *Guardian* article, John Hooper tells the story of two German murderers and devil worshippers, Manuela and Daniel Ruda, who progressed from involvement in a 'gothic club' to bloodsucking, graveyard parties and eventually murder.[4]

In one typical article, Gerald Wright and Stuart Millar highlight Harris and Klebold's membership of Goth subculture claiming that, "central to the Trenchcoat Mafia's identity was their association with 'dark metal' Goth music."[5] The article quotes several song lyrics from Harris' website, implying that Harris followed the 'instructions' in the songs. The piece concludes with a reference to 'backward messages' in songs by Marilyn Manson. The 'urban myth' of backward tracks encouraging teenage violence has existed at least since the 1970s and has no more basis in reality than it did then. Furthermore, it is hard to see why Manson would conceal 'subliminal' messages in his songs when his lyrics blatantly emphasise evil and death. Most of these articles construct the link between Goth and violence as taken-for-granted common sense, sometimes providing 'expert' opinion to validate the notion that Goths are emotionally disturbed or vulnerable to the influence of religious cults.[6]

Many Christian websites also perpetuate the view that Goth music and Pagan religions are dangerous and evil. Several make links between Goth or rock music, Satanism and murder. In relation to Paganism, one site asks, "what is the difference between witchcraft and Satanism? Both are anti-Christ by definition … Both are forbidden in the Holy Scriptures"[7] Such websites include Biblical quotes linked to passages from presumably 'Pagan' books, including 'Harry Potter', and often feature statements from 'former witches' who provide 'expert testimony' based on their knowledge of Paganism and the danger that it poses: "I used to be a white witch … I had my own pack of tarot cards that I did readings from, I was a clairvoyant medium, did séances, astrology, palm reading and had a witches' spell book … I know now that the world is being deceived by this witchcraft/new age stuff."[8] The author of this e-mail constructs herself as an expert with personal experience of being a dedicated witch, before stating that she now sees the risk involved in such activities.

Paganism and witchcraft are depicted in many factual books as well as fictional texts, films and TV programmes. These portrayals vary, but some make the link between Paganism and demonic forces. The film *The Craft* for example, revolves around teenage girls invoking dangerous powers and harming others through witchcraft. The media takes a dualistic view of Goths and Pagans: they are either evil and dangerous, or eccentric, strange and pathetic. Jonathan Elcock points out that people who participate in role-play games are portrayed similarly by the media: as either menacing and satanic, or geeks with poor social skills.[9] In all three cases there is an implicit assumption that those drawn to role-play, Goth music or Paganism, are somewhat innately pathetic or weird and therefore vulnerable to the 'evil side' of the subculture.

B. Past Research on Youth Subcultures
Social psychological research on subcultures has concentrated on the relationship between individual identity and group identity The social psychological rationale most often applied to this area is 'social identity theory'.[10] This suggests that people organise how they perceive themselves and others by categorising themselves into groups and then identifying with one group as opposed to another. Our sense of self-esteem comes from how we evaluate *our* group in relation to *other* groups. Research by H. Tajfel and J. C. Turner has found that people accentuate the similarities between members of their group and exaggerate the differences between themselves and members of other groups. They also tend to maximise their advantage in relation to others, thus enhancing the identity and esteem of their group members. Social identity theory however, has been criticised for its failure to be applied outside western culture.[11] A related approach is Roy F. Baumeister's 'myth of pure evil'.[12] His work is useful for examining subcultures like Goth and Paganism,

which may be persecuted to some extent by other groups. Baumeister suggests that when we are attacked by others we tend to portray our group - 'us' - as purely good and innocent and the other group - 'them' - as chaotic, sadistic and motiveless. I will draw on these theories to some extent in order to examine how Goths and Pagans use 'us and them' classifications to describe their experiences.

Sue Widdicombe states that previous research on youth subcultures ignores the way in which group members understand the significance and meaning of their subculture.[13] She suggests that this can be overcome through discourse analysis, a technique that examines how people use language to construct versions of their experiences, rather than assuming that language simply reflects internal attitudes or 'true' events. Discourse analysis concentrates on the way in which people draw on cultural or linguistic resources to construct their conversations in ways that will produce a desired effect. This method is employed below. It is a social constructionist approach which involves reading and re-reading interview transcripts, and then noting the common themes that emerge and examining how interviewees use language to construct their accounts, for example as factual and/or persuasive.

C. The Current Research

Unlike many of the members of youth subcultures previously studied in sociological and social psychological literature, Goths and Pagans are not necessarily male or working-class. Most of the interviewees in this research were women, only two (pseudonyms Adam and Gerald), were male, but there seems to be roughly equal numbers of male and female Goths and Pagans, possibly even more females than males, within the Pagan movement. The interviewees were all tertiary students from working and middle-class families of varying religious backgrounds. All were between eighteen and twenty-five, although it should be pointed out that Goths are not confined to this age group and Paganism is certainly not considered a 'youth' subculture. I wanted to explore the accounts of younger Pagans since they seem to be the prime demographic for texts on this topic. Previous work in this area has unfortunately been limited to studies on older Pagans who grew up in the 1960s.[14]

All the interviewees were known to me through mutual friends prior to this research. Although my analysis is necessarily rooted in the relationships that I had built up with the interviewees, I have maintained enough 'analytical distance' to make the study a viable representation of the wider Goth and Pagan communities.[15] The interviews lasted for approximately sixty minutes each and were conducted on a one-to-one basis with the exception of my conversations with Gerald and Carrie (pseudonyms). Interviewees were asked general questions about their background, the way in which they defined themselves, how they came to Goth/Paganism, their understanding of their group's history, and the way they felt other people perceived them. In addition to these interviews I also obtained some shorter interview transcripts from another study on Goths identity that had been carried out by a student who I was supervising at the time.[16] Combining this data meant that there were nine interviewees altogether. Eight of these were Goths, three of whom were also Pagan, and the other interviewee was a non-Goth Pagan. Several of the Goths who did not define themselves as Pagan did express interest in alternative religions.

Discourse analysis transcriptions can look strange to those unfamiliar with them. This is because they faithfully record the way people speak, including every 'um' and 'er'. As a code for the reader, commas indicate a pause. **Bold** text was said with emphasis. Anything in square brackets [ ] is a note that has been added during transcription. Some of the minimal prompts used by the interviewers to encourage the subjects to continue have been removed, for example 'mm', 'yeah', 'mmhm'. This is to make quotes more readable. Such prompts can be seen as the verbal equivalent of nods and other body language which could not be recorded.

It is important to note that the aim of this research is not to question the truthfulness or validity of the accounts of the subjects. Rather, this study seeks to understand how the various accounts are constructed and what is gained from these constructions. Discourse analysis assumes that people are performing social 'actions' when they use language, that is, they justify, explain, defend or persuade, it is therefore important to consider what actions their dialogue achieves and what potential arguments it is designed to counteract.[17] This is not to say that people consciously construct their arguments in a deceptive or manipulative way in order to be persuasive, but rather that tacit or common-sense communicative skills are employed by speakers to construct their accounts as factual and legitimate.[18]

2.   Analysis: 'You's All Satanists'
Many themes emerged through the discourse analysis of my interview transcripts. The one I will focus on here is how Goths and Pagans felt themselves to be negatively perceived and how they responded to these perceptions. In order to make the analysis as clear as possible I will impose this loose structure:
A. Negative perceptions
B. Who is prejudiced?
C. Responding to prejudice
D. Understanding prejudice

Discourses of other-ness and group history will also be drawn out in the analysis as these issues recurred throughout the interviews.

A. Negative Perceptions
All the Goths and Pagans interviewed agreed that people outside their subculture labelled them as evil or Satanic. Indeed when asked how others responded to them, many of the Pagans immediately said the word 'Satanist'. Most of the Goths described being labelled as 'freaks'. Rather than being explicitly labelled as Satanists, most of them spoke of being seen as a 'witch' and went on to say that witches were often confused with Satanists. Some also said that people were suspicious that they might have an evil or corrupting influence on others, particularly children.

Most of the interviewees gave specific examples from personal experience to support these statements. Daisy and Nikki both related times when people have responded to their Pentagrams: a five-pointed star enclosed by a circle, often worn as jewellery by both Pagans and Goths.

Nikki
The symbol of the pentagram, um, which people, when they see it they automatically think, 'oo Satanism'... er coz, um, one of my other friends, he um, went to get a tattoo, last year ... and he wanted a pentagram, and he went into the, tattoo parlour and the guy said 'oh you're a Satanist are you' (laughs) and he was like **'no**, I am **not** thank-you'
[Interviewer says: yeah, so it's really common]
yeah, and I, I used to draw them as well just as like, doodling at school I'd just draw pentagrams and this girl came up to you and she was like 'oo are you a Satanist Nikki that's the sign of the devil' and (laughs) I just thought, 'no'.

Daisy
Always worn a pentagram ring ... and, people have always looked at it and gone 'oo ooo Satanism' [dumb voice] 'no, no', ... and er, yeah, I've often had, yeah, certainly in, during my GCSEs and my A levels I had to defend my myself against allegations, and the whole of Paganism against 'ay you's all Satanists though aren't you' [dumb voice] most people are absolutely pig ignorant about it

It is interesting that both Nikki and Daisy use the same wording in their examples: 'oo Satanism'. This is known as active voicing: the reporting of speech within accounts.[19] It is unlikely that words reported like this were originally spoken exactly as they are presented. Daisy probably cannot remember perfectly back to her schooldays and Nikki was not even present in the tattoo parlour. So there is some reason why utterances reported in this way are designed to be heard *as if* they were said at the time.[20] Here is seems that active voicing is used to show that these events really happened, in support of the claim that people often see Pagans as Satanic.

Both Daisy and Nikki also use hypothetical illustration.[21] They distil recurrent features from actual events into one hypothetical example: someone coming up to them in school and saying 'oo are you a Satanist?' or 'ay you's all Satanists though aren't you'. This prevents direct examination because it is not one real-life event. It also gives the impression that events like this have happened many times. It is clear that the interviewer picks up on this in the comment after Nikki's tattoo story: 'so it's really common'.

Finally, the active voicing used here highlights the prejudices of those speaking. Later on both Nikki and Daisy spend a lot of time explaining why the notion that Pagans are Satanists is wrong. Here they accomplish a similar thing without needing any explanation. They simply put on a dumb or silly voice when imitating the people in their stories, so it is obvious that they regard these perceptions as ridiculous. Daisy's example is particularly clear because her active voicing is filtered with poor English: 'you's all Satanists', implying that people with such prejudices are generally 'pig ignorant'.

The Pagan interviewees tended to depict the prejudice they had experienced as ignorant and annoying since it meant that they were not taken seriously or treated with respect. They did not however, describe aggressive attacks in the way that the Goths did. The Goths all mentioned that abuse was shouted at them from the street, whereas the Pagans tended to relate examples of prejudice in one-to-one situations with people they knew. It seems likely that the physical 'look' of Goths, a major part of their culture, is one reason for this distanced abuse, Pagans are not as easy to recognise. Perhaps this is why many of the Pagans' stories are about people noticing their pentagrams: one aspect of their appearance that hints at their beliefs.

Like the Pagans, the Goths used specific examples to support the claim that they experienced prejudice. Gerald in particular told several long stories of occasions when people were violent toward him. The overall picture was of regular verbal abuse that frequently became physical.

Gerald
I mean, up, up here at one point last year there was, when
we were walking up [road name] there was about, twenty,
odd people up there who just started yelling random stuff
and one guy decided he was gonna come down and try and
do something about he ended up trying a leap up and hit me
round the head with a beer can.

Georgina
I mean I've sat in the pub before with a bunch of blokes we
all had leather jackets on all dressed in black erm all the
blokes had long hair and apparently (laughs) we'd been
staring at people as if we wanted a fight and I mean this
was a bunch of what I'd definitely determine as normals ...
and it was **us** that calmed the situation down the others
were up for a fight and whatever but we said, 'no look mate
don't wanna fight we're just sitting here we're really sorry
if we were staring' or something I mean none of us actually
had registered they were even in the pub (laughs) you
know.

Here it seems that Georgina, Gerald and Carrie all construct themselves as
reasonable people in unreasonable situations. Georgina and Gerald both
tell their stories in a format that Robin Wooffitt refers to as 'I was just X
... when Y'.[22] They set the scene of their group doing something normal
and everyday, sitting in the pub or walking up a particular road, when they
were verbally attacked by a group of 'normals' or 'drunks'. Wooffitt says
that this type of discourse generally emphasises the normality of the
situation and speaker in relation to the strangeness and abnormality of
what happened to them. In this case, Georgina, Gerald and Carrie's
accounts serve to construct their groups as reasonable people, in relation to
the non-Goths who react in shocking and unreasonable ways. Georgina
underlines the unreasonableness of the 'normals' thinking they were being
stared at, with her statement that 'none of us actually had registered they
were even in the pub'. This is what G. Jefferson refers to as a 'normalising
device': the speaker's way of emphasising that they are an 'ordinary
person' who reacted in a normal way to events.[23]

Following the quote given here, Gerald and Carrie went on to
further construct themselves as reasonable by attempting to excuse the
behaviour of their attackers (drunkenness, or the external fact that Gerald
was already having a 'bad week' for abuse). They even seemed to take on
some responsibility by saying that they 'should've ignored them more than

we did'. However, they then saw their slight retaliation as reasonable since both of them found that they could not predict whether ignoring the abuse would have helped or made it worse. This further illustrates the random, chaotic nature of the attacks that they experienced and can be read in relation to Baumeister's myth of pure evil: the common way in which people construct themselves - 'us' as good, innocent victims provoked by 'them', the sadistic, chaotic attackers.[24]

B. Who is Prejudiced?
When interviewees were talking about those who were prejudiced, they mostly said 'people' or 'they' to indicate that people in general are ignorant. Both groups felt that society perceives them negatively. This suggests that the interviewees constructed themselves as 'outside' mainstream culture. This construction comes across when the Goths and Pagans talk about the groups who are prejudiced against them - the same groups that they construct themselves in relation to. The Goths mostly talk about 'norms' or mainstream people, whereas the Pagans talk about Christians because they view Christianity as the most dominant religious system in the UK. In both cases, the interviewees spoke against the structured 'rules' inherent in mainstream fashion/music or Christianity. The idea is that their group is open-minded and varied, whereas the other group is structured and unthinkingly follow established codes of behaviour. Similar comparisons were made by those involved in rave culture in Jonathan Elcock and Yvonne Adair's study, where rave culture was contrasted with the judgmental mainstream and beer-oriented, lecherous pub culture.[25] The constructions of the interviewees could be explained by social identity theory: we see those within our own group as individuals, and those in the other group as all the same.[26] Later quotes in this section however, suggest that interviewees' accounts were somewhat more complex than this.

Georgina
> There are the more townie normals that I just really don't get on with because they have the view that you must dress like this you must wear all the named brands you must like clubby music erm.

Su
> Um I view people who dress in a conformist way as very, easily, um, as, very, easy to blend in people that kind of don't think for themselves people who, take the kind of easy option and, simply, wear what they're told to wear

rather than thinking for themselves um.

Examples of Goths defining themselves favourably in contrast to the norm can also be seen in the earlier quotes where Gerald, Carrie and Georgina construct 'normals' as violent and less intelligent than themselves.

The Pagan interviewees generally spent time showing that they had some experience of Christianity, from home or school, and then talked about it being restrictive, structured and intolerant in comparison to Paganism.

Nikki
And I, I preferred their, sort of rule system that, the only thing they have is, just, harm none, which I think is fair enough rather than having the, 'thou shalt not kill thou shalt not covet thy neighbour's, donkey or' (laughs) it gets a bit far fetched that.

Christine
I, liked that fact that it was so, laid back and relaxed, really, and that it meant that you didn't have to, um, be, talking about your religion all the time saying 'oh I, I, believe in Jesus' or 'I'm, I go to church every Sunday' or whatever, you don't have to do that.

They also stated that Paganism is more concerned with the environment and less patriarchal than Christianity. They used historical references to implicate Christianity in persecution, control, oppression and money-making, in contrast to Paganism which has always been natural and free.

I found tensions in many of the interviews when it came to notions of tolerance. On one hand most participants expressed intolerance of those who abused them, or members of their group who gave them a bad name, on the other hand they were wary of sounding intolerant themselves, particularly because many of them saw tolerance as a big part of the Goth and Pagan ideology and also because they had personally experienced intolerance. Although many of the Goth interviewees spoke about unintelligent, aggressive 'normals' or 'trendies', some of them were uncomfortable about labelling people in this way. Adam expressed this view most strongly when he was asked about so-called 'normals'.

Adam
I **don't** like that word at all, erm, it distinguishes between things too much, I don't see things as having black and

white boundaries i.e. you're **this** or you're **that**, I think
things exist in a far more fluid state, I know plenty of
people who look perfectly normal, erm, and I get on with
them **really** well, they've got a lot of similar interests to
me, erm, and I don't think it's fair to use that word **at all**, in
what way is it referring to them as normal, is it normal in
appearance, normal in intelligence, mind set, then you get
into the whole run of things, what is a normal state of
mind?

Georgina however, justified her labelling of 'norms' by talking of them as
a dominant social group who also label her. She therefore rationalised that
it was reasonable for her to label them, but it is clear that she considers
this issue to be problematic.

> **Georgina**
> Erm so I mean we're not **really** being offensive when we
> call people norms it's just a way of defining people I
> suppose I mean they'd call me a Goth and I'd call them a
> norm because there isn't actually a sort of subculture or
> whatever that **they** are part of erm
> [Interviewer asks: because they're part of the bigger
> culture?]
> Yeah they're part of what's meant to be sort of your general
> English culture so they're norms.
> [Interviewer asks: So you're allowed to label them as well]
> yeah I think so I think if they label us then we can label
> them back

Many of the Pagan interviewees mentioned Christians that they knew who
did not fit into any of their negative preconceptions. Again, this may serve
to show that Pagans are aware that the 'us and them' distinction is not as
simple as they might have at first thought. It also positions them as even
more reasonable, thoughtful and tolerant, in comparison to the 'other'
group.

C. Responding to Prejudice
During the interviews most people spent some time countering the
assumptions that they felt were made about them. The Pagans used two
main devices to challenge the claim that they were evil or satanic. The first
was to show that Paganism was staunchly opposed to causing harm. All

the Pagan interviewees said that the main rule of Paganism was not to hurt anyone.

Christine

Pagans don't do that though [try to harm others], if you, if someone actually does like start, doing curses or whatever that person, couldn't be classed as a Pagan because they have the harm none thing.

Christine, like the other Pagan interviewees, cites the 'harm none' rule to show that 'real' Pagans could not be involved in evil in the way that they are portrayed by outsiders. She goes so far as to say that someone who did this could not be Pagan.

Daisy and Christine also both spend some time explaining how Paganism is very different to Satanism. Daisy takes the view that Satanism is negative, dangerous and ridiculous. In contrast, Christine expresses the view that Satanism is fine as a belief system, but it is just not her belief system. When Ann talks about not being satanic or evil, she incorporates both the previously mentioned devices into her speech. First, she has very different beliefs to Satanists, and second she is non-violent:

Ann

I just say well 'I can't be a Satanist I don't believe in god, you can't have one without the other, therefore, I'm not a Satanist, so', but they don't seem to **get** it (laughs) … I used to get approached by the god squad quite a lot … and, sometimes they'd come up on their own and have a go at us and say 'oi, you, you're going to burn in hell you witch', and I'd just confront them and say 'well, how can you say that you don't actually **know** me', you know it, does annoy me a lot because, I mean I am, like a, I'm basically, I'm quite a gentle person, I'm not actually that violent, I don't **steal**, I don't do **drugs** I, certainly don't you know, go, robbing things and bashing old ladies and taking heroin.

Here Ann uses two three-part lists to illustrate how different she is from the assumptions made about her by 'the God squad'. Jefferson says that a three-part list is a culturally available resource for list construction which we often use in everyday conversation.[27] Here Ann starts with a general three part list and then builds on it with a list of three more specific examples: 'I'm not … that violent … I don't steal … I don't do drugs' and then: 'I … don't go robbing things and bashing old ladies and taking heroin'. Listing these behaviours together indicates a broader class of activities that Ann does not do, backing up her contention that she is 'gentle' and not evil or criminal in any way. By listing these behaviours together Ann also makes the point that the assumption made about her group is that they are generally bad in many ways. The extreme examples specifically serve to refute these assumptions.

The Goth interviewees also spent some time countering the idea that they are evil, violent or dangerous. Georgina's story about 'normals' in a pub trying to start a fight, constructs her group as peaceful and the others as violent. Gerald uses a similar story to disprove the idea that Goths are violent.

Gerald

Um, again this is, something someone else has said to me um, they were, so wherever, wherever it was they came from they had, sort of a club, well basically there was sort of your typical dancey club, on one side of the road and, an alternative metal club on the other side, on one night and um, invariably every, every night when the clubs kicked out the police would show up, and end up arresting loads of people, and, they'd always arrest, all the metallers, and stuff, and, this regardless of who's fault it was, and in, in the um, police van as they drove them back coz they never, actually, um prosecuted they would just drive them to the station let them go, and so this person goes, 'why is it you always arrest us you, never actually, sort of, prosecute or anything you just literally drive to the station and let us go again', the policeman turned round and said 'coz that's what the public expect to see'.

Gerald begins this story quite vaguely: he does not know where the club was, and defines the storyteller as 'someone else'. At the end of the story however, he uses active voicing, even though it is unlikely that either he or the person who told him the story could remember exactly what was said. This active voicing clearly displays that even the policeman is aware that the public perception of alternative 'metallers' as violent, is wrong. This could be seen as an externalising device, since it puts words into the mouth of a policeman, someone in authority with experience of violence. [28] The story also suggests that it would be easier for the policeman to accept the public perception of metallers as violent, since this would accord with him taking them to the station. The fact that he admits the true reason for his actions makes his statement even stronger and more likely to be accurate.

Speaking about prejudice often led the interviewees to question whether they dressed as they did 'for attention' or 'to get a reaction'. It seems that they were countering a discourse often used against them: that they are only Goth in order to get a reaction or that the Goth appearance is attention-seeking. Georgina and Gerald both counter this argument by stating that they get more reactions from people they know when they wear non-Goth clothing. Carrie and Su both admit that to some degree they do like getting a response from people, but they argue that this is not the only reason they do it. They have received attention from people because of being Goth and they have decided that they might as well see it positively.

When talking about coping with prejudice, Su, Carrie, Gerald and Nikki all admitted that they partly aimed to get a reaction from people by dressing as they did. At other points, they suggest that their Goth clothes divert attention from other aspects of their appearance. Georgina used dark clothes to disguise her tallness. In her case dark clothes enabled her to fade into the background. Gerald may have done something similar. He likes the fact people are commenting on something he can change rather than something he cannot. Carrie says that one reason she wears Goth clothes is so that people attend to them rather than to her weight. Therefore the clothes are worn to 'get a reaction', but she only wants this reaction to prevent people responding to her in the way that they used to when she was in school.

Georgina
Yeah so I'd just go for nondescript clothes and black was just sort of pretty nondescript really (laughs) erm and **then** I mean people then started calling me a Goth cos I'd always wear black.

Gerald and Carrie
Carrie: I think that, certainly w, you know when I was in school and when I, had um, when I was being bullied quite a lot, um, it was to do with my appearance, and, you know being, fat or being, ugly or whatever um, and then, when I, now that I wear this sort of stuff, I know that if I'm walking down a street, most people don't have time to think anything more than, 'she's a Goth' or, 'she's a freak' or, and that sort of, negative, thoughts I can deal with a whole lot better than them thinking that I'm fat.
Gerald: They they they're commenting on something that you can go home and change, out of, it's something that

you can literally change and, be, I dunno **normal**, by, literally almost clicking your fingers.

D. Understanding Prejudice

Interviewees also spent some time trying to explain and understand the assumptions made about them. The Goth interviewees explained the prejudice they experienced in three main ways: the fact that Goths are not part of the 'social norm', the insecurity/fear on the part of their abusers, or their desire to 'look good'.

Ann

I do feel, I mean obviously being Goth you kind of get rejected don't you, aren't part of the social norm.

Gerald

I always say they're just, looking for something to sort of, put themselves one up on, their mates and stuff, so, it's weird, I always, sort of justify in my head some kind of in, feriority complex, they're always, coz they're not, secure in the group or something and they just need to try and, show off say look 'I've done, this' and all the rest of it.

Gerald also states that people are 'invariably scared by what they don't understand' and Adam suggests an element of homophobia in people responding negatively to Goths, since male Goths dress up and wear make-up.

Carrie also constructs prejudice against her group as seemingly more acceptable than other types of prejudice since she *chooses* to be Goth.

Carrie

Yeah I think it's it's, much more accepted as well, it's **OK** for them, to do this to us because we made the choice to dress like this, that's what it comes down to.

Gerald and Carrie go on to argue that prejudice against Goths is seen as more acceptable than homophobia or racism because of this element of choice. This issue of whether Goth identity is 'natural' or an option, came up several times. The assumption here is that prejudice is less acceptable when it is directed at people who have no choice about their appearance or lifestyle. This echoes discourses about sexuality: some anti-gay campaigners argue that homosexuality is a choice and some gay-rights activists counter that it is an 'innate' condition. A strong discourse in

Western culture at present seems to be that biologically determined behaviour is somehow more 'real' than behaviour that is the product of socialisation or cultural expectations. Some of the interviewees argued that being Goth is not something that they can help since it is the only way that they are able to feel comfortable or 'right'. This discourse counters the claim, and the prejudice attached to it, that Goth identity is chosen.

> *Gerald and Carrie*
> Gerald: walking back yesterday in that light blue shirt and stuff from work I felt like a right tit, I feel **so** awkward just, wandering around it's just, it does feel **wrong** on me, which is bizarre most people th, just don't understand that, as a concept and stuff but, it just, feels awkward it doesn't feel right, I sort of, I mean when I went down for the interview actually I mean I saw a reflection of myself in, in um, sort of window wearing exactly the same and I didn't recognise myself, there was a couple of seconds before I twigged it was actually **me**, and stuff so
> Carrie: yeah I I, totally understand that coz um, when I went to [holiday abroad] last year, and, it was, really too hot to wear what I'd normally wear, um, so, I had to change to wearing green sort of kaki type stuff and, you know a few, a few years before, I did wear, quite a lot of, of kaki but um, it just, didn't feel **right** and, once I'd, um, once I got to [city] and I tried on, some, stuff in a, in a Goth, fetish type, store I really, didn't wanna take it off again, coz, it just, it does feel wrong and I just feel I look very unattractive wearing, that as well, coz that's just, I don't know it's weird but.
> Gerald: there was no sort of **conscious** decision involved there.

Georgina also talks about being comfortable in Goth clothes, and the feelings of anxiety she experienced when her mother would not let her wear them. Overall the Goth interviewees, when contemplating a future identity, often felt that they could not easily dress in any other way. Many said that they have tried to fit in with the mainstream and failed, often at school. This failure is presented as another reason why they could not be anything other than *other*.

Like the Goths, the Pagan interviewees explained the prejudice against them in terms of general ignorance and the fear of difference. They spent some time exploring prejudice in historical terms, placing responsibility on early Christians who labelled Pagans as 'evil'. Ann, Daisy and Nikki all describe how early Christians renamed the Pagan god Pan as Satan. They argue that this was a clever ploy to convert Pagans to Christianity and see contemporary accusations of child sacrifice as a similar technique used by Christians to demonise Pagans. As in previous quotes, the interviewees depict Christianity as authoritarian, structured and hierarchical, in stark opposition to the free and open nature of Paganism.

Ann
Witchcraft isn't really linked to Satanism
[Interviewer asks: so why did, why do people make that connection]
the church, when they came over to this country they said 'right then, you're a Satanist' because um, Satan is **Pan**, anyway so he's he's a major Pagan god, um, so that's where they get it from it it's just bred into people, people just think, that's what it is now because, I mean the church did a good job of it then really didn't they, I mean if you're going to come over what's the best sales pitch ever, say 'what you're doing now, paganism is, evil, and that you're all gonna, **burn** for eternity for believing in that so believe **ours** instead and give us money, and you'll be alright' (laughs).

All the Pagans traced their religion to ancient roots. In the Pagan interviews, the subjects draw on a wider social discourse which assumes that a traceable history confers authenticity. Such an argument is often used for example, by those in favour of meat-eating or fox-hunting. Like 'scientific' approaches, the discourse of 'antiquity' serves to justify and legitimise beliefs or behaviour.

One fascinating aspect of this discourse was the way in which interviewees told the history of Paganism as the story of a group of persecuted outsiders. This echoes the stories they tell about their own harassment. It seems that the historical discourse legitimises their experiences, making them part of a group who have suffered for centuries. This sense of connection may also help to justify their present group commitment. Interviewees make comparisons between witch-burning and the Jewish holocaust and between the Christian taking of Pagan holy sites and white Australians claiming land ownership of sites sacred to aboriginal peoples. These links serve to construct Pagans as a group who have a right to redress after years of persecution.

3.   Conclusions: 'The Other Society'

My interviews with Goths and Pagans identified many similarities between the two groups. All the interviewees said that they were perceived to be Satanic, evil or freakish. Both Goths and Pagans were also aware of their role as 'outsiders' and spoke about prejudice from 'people' and 'them'. The interviewees identified themselves as outside the 'mainstream' and the 'norm', which they generally understood to be rule-governed, inflexible and intolerant, whilst their group in contrast, was free, open-minded and accepting. The Goths generally constructed their identities as other to 'normal' people of their age who followed fashion and trendy music. The Pagans distinguished their religion from Christianity, which they saw as part of mainstream culture. It appears that members of both groups have responded to accusations of 'otherness' and 'difference' by embracing these qualities in a positive way. This process is evident in both the personal and group histories told by the interviewees.

The idea of otherness involved some interesting contradictions. When relating experiences of prejudice, the interviewees often used 'normalising devices', constructing themselves as 'ordinary people' under attack.[29] At other points they saw the 'norm' as something they wished to avoid. Such behaviour is characteristic of the general population: most of us use different rhetorical devices at different times when trying to create specific effects.[30] The discourse of being an 'everyday person' encourages other people to sympathise with our situation, whereas the discourse of being 'different' emphasises our individuality and uniqueness. Another aspect of otherness that the interviewees had to negotiate, was the possible criticism that they were being intolerant or making assumptions about 'norms' or 'the mainstream'. Most of them either justified this by using phrases such as 'they label us' and 'they are the dominant group in society'. Alternatively, many mentioned that they had friends who were normal or Christian. It appears then, that the idea of otherness is a major theme in the way that the members of both groups construct their identity. It is not surprising that Su and Adam, two of the Goth interviewees, have set up a group at their college called 'the other society'.

Notes

1.   Chesters, 2001.
2.   For example, Busman, 1990, 38; Sullivan, 1990, 24.
3.   Smith, 1999, 12.
4.   Hooper, 2002, 2
5.   Wright and Millar, 2002.
6.   Elcock, 2001, 1-4.

7. Brown, 2002.
8. Madrak and Madrak, 2002.
9. Elcock, 2001, 1-4.
10. Tajfel and Turner, 1979, 33-47.
11. Wetherell, 1996, 217.
12. Baumeister, 1996, 17-18.
13. Widdecombe, 1993 94-114.
14. For example Kemp, 1993.
15. Elcock and Adair, 1996, 4.
16. Chesters.
17. Edwards and Potter, 1992, 2-3.
18. Wooffitt, 1992, 2.
19. Ibid.,155-188.
20. Hutchby and Wooffitt, 1998, 225-227.
21. Wooffitt, 84-85.
22. Ibid., 117-155.
23. Jefferson, 1984.
24. Baumeister, 68-69.
25. Elcock and Adair, 11-12.
26. Tajfel and Turner, 33-47.
27. Jefferson, 1991.
28. Edwards and Potter, 104-108.
29. Jefferson, 1984.
30. Potter, 1996, 119-175.

References

Baumeister, R. F. (1996), *Evil: Inside Human Violence and Cruelty.* New York: W. H. Freeman.

Brown, D. L. (20 February, 2002), 'Logos Resource Page'. www.logosresourcepages.org/pagen.html.

Bussman, J. (20 February, 2002), 'Glastonbury Festival: The drapes of Goths.' *Guardian,* 26th June: 38. 1990. The Guardian Website. http://www.guardian.co.uk

Chesters, S. (2001), 'Outcasts and Freaks: An ethnographic discourse analysis of subcultural influences and motivations.' Unpublished undergraduate manuscript towards psychology degree. University of Gloucestershire. UK.

Edwards, D. and J. Potter (1992), *Discursive Psychology.* London: Sage.

Elcock, J. (2001), 'Fantasy worlds: Constructions of role-playing games.' Unpublished paper. School of Social Sciences. University of Gloucestershire. UK.

Elcock, J. and Y. Adair (1996), 'It's not just the drugs'. Unpublished paper. School of Social Sciences. University of Gloucestershire. UK.

Fleming, A. (director) (1996) *The Craft* [film]. Columbia Pictures. USA.

Hooper, J. (2002), 'Blood-drinking devil worshippers face life for ritual Satanic killing'. *Guardian,* 2nd February. 2.

Hutchby, I. and R. Wooffitt (1998), *Conversation Analysis.* Cambridge: Polity Press.

Jefferson, G. (1984), ' "At first I thought": a normalizing device for extraordinary events.' Unpublished manuscript. Katholieke Hogeschool Tilburg.

Jefferson, G. (1991), 'List construction as a task and a resource', in: G. Psathas and R. Frankel (eds.) *Interactional Competence.* Hillsdale, NJ: Lawrence Erlbaum Associates.

Kemp, A. (1993), *Witchcraft and Paganism Today.* London: Brockhampton Press.

Madrak, S. and E. Madrak, (20 February, 2002), 'Demonbuster.com'. www.demonbuster.com

Potter, J. (1996), 'Attitudes, social representations and discursive psychology', in: M. Wetherell (ed.) *Identities, Groups and Social Issues,* Milton Keynes: OU Press. 119-175.

Smith, A. (1999), 'Have you goth what it takes?'. *Sunday Times,* 9th May, Culture. 12.

Sullivan, C. (1990), 'Black capes, death fixations, Shelley recitals and an infinite supply of doom and gloom'. *Guardian,* 26th July. 24.

Tajfel, H. and J.C. Turner (1979), 'An integrative theory of intergroup conflict', in: G. W. Austin and S. Worchel (eds.) *The Social Psychology of Intergroup Relations*. Montery, California: Brooks/Cole. 33-47.

Wetherell, M. (ed.) (1996), *Identities, Groups and Social Issues*. Milton Keynes: OU Press.

Whitworth, D. (1999), 'Gloomy tribal craze that was born in Britain.' *Times,* 22nd April. 5.

Widdecombe, S. (1993), 'Autobiography and change: rhetoric and authenticity of 'Gothic' style', in: E. Burman and I. Parker (eds.) *Discoursing Analytic Research: Repertoires and Readings of Texts in Action,* London: Routledge. 94-114.

Wooffitt, R. (1992), *Telling Tales of the Unexpected.* Hemel Hempstead: Harvester Wheatsheaf.

Wright, G. and S. Millar (20 February, 2002), 'A clique within a clique, obsessed with guns, death and Hitler.' *Guardian,* April 22nd. 1999. The Guardian Website.
http://www.guardian.co.uk/Archive/Article/0,4273,3856954,00.html,

The Evils of Christianization:
A Pagan Perspective on European History

Michael F. Strmiska

Any thoughtful student of history soon comes to understand that major events affecting large numbers of people can be approached and assessed from a variety of angles and perspectives. It is a durable truism that 'history is written by the victors,' with many historical accounts of previous times slanted to favour the interests of particular nations or social groups over others less privileged. In recent times, social and intellectual trends such as feminism, deconstructionism, postcolonialism and indigenous people's movements, have raised awareness of the importance of acknowledging the voices and viewpoints of persons, groups and nations who have been ignored or devalued in history as it has been construed, constructed and promulgated by the dominant social groups of past times.

The change of religions that took place in Europe when Christianity spread beyond the confines of the Roman Empire replacing the traditional, nature-oriented, 'Pagan' religions of other parts of Europe, is arguably one of the major historical transformations in European history.[1] By and large, in the transition from Paganism to Christianity, it has been assumed that Christian domination and suppression of pre-existing Pagan traditions, was a natural and necessary thing.[2]

This account of European history, grounded in dogmatic convictions that view Christianity as superior to other religions, has a long and venerable history in its own right, beginning with the Christian scriptures themselves. To Medieval participants in this Christian-centred discourse, European civilization was the same as 'Christendom.' Even today, it is still commonplace to refer to Europe as the 'Christian West.' In the last two centuries however, the authority of this paradigm or metanarrative of Christian supremacy, has been corroded by the general secularization of Western societies, and by West's increasing contact with, and knowledge of, other world religions.

The deflation of this metanarrative of Christian privilege has enormous implications for the position of Christianity in relation to other religions in our increasingly pluralistic societies, and equally important ramifications for how we view and interpret the past. With the paradigm of unquestioned Christian supremacy giving way to a new ideal of religious tolerance and coexistence in which religious pluralism is viewed as the norm, we have reason to look with new eyes at the transition from

Paganism to Christianity in Europe.

This change of religions is often characterized as the 'rise' of Christianity, but it should also be understood as the 'fall' of Paganism in Europe: a fall which was neither simple nor painless, but a bloody and protracted struggle. Christianity did not simply 'rise' - it conquered. Nor did Paganism merely 'fall' - it was crushed. The temples of the old religions in Europe did not simply collapse - they were torn down by Christians, and in some cases, recycled as building materials for the construction of Christian churches.

In many areas, the adherents of Pagan religions fought tenaciously to preserve their ancestral traditions, even if their struggles were ultimately in vain and their traditions so nearly obliterated that only the most fragmentary traces remained. Clearly there were, and are, two sides to this story, but we usually only hear from the side which celebrates the victory of Christianity. What would we hear were we to listen to the voices of the Pagans who suffered loss, defeat and erasure? What would we find were we to analyse these past peoples and their religions, rather than dismiss them?

I believe that the most basic and important lesson from such research and contemplation, is to realise that religious pluralism - a lively clash of competing Pagan and Christian religious cultures - existed in Medieval Europe 1,000 years ago. According to Russian theorist Bakhtin, an active religious *heteroglossia* or religious *dialogue* certainly existed.[3] This dialogue ended with the victory of Christian monologue and mono-logic. This monologue however, never succeeded entirely in eradicating all traces of Paganism, which lived on in folklore, popular customs and celebrations, and even infiltrated Christianity itself via Pagan gods remade into Christian saints or reviled as forms of the Christian devil, and holy days reinterpreted as feast days for Christian saints.

In understanding that Pagan religion represented another distinct dimension of European life, both before, during and after Christianization, a more nuanced and multi-dimensional understanding of European history and culture can be realised. In the complexity of our modern world, it is important to acknowledge that the forces of Christianization were continually striving to impose religious uniformity and erase even the memory of religious dialogue and pluralism.

In the following brief case-studies, which looks at the roles played by the Holy Roman Emperor Charlemagne, and the Scandinavian Vikings, during the religious conflicts between Pagans and Christians in Medieval Europe, I will attempt to show how examining European history from the Pagan point of view, illuminates important issues and raises valuable questions for our contemporary understanding of the past.

1.   Reconsidering Charlemagne

The reign of the Frankish king and later Holy Roman Emperor Charlemagne, is often viewed as one of the milestones in the establishment of European Christian civilization. In recent times, with the increasing strength of pan-European institutions in the framework of the European Union, Charlemagne is seen as an early herald of European unity.[4] His rule is often praised as a 'Carolingian renaissance' for fostering arts and learning within institutions of the Christian church. There are however, other dimensions of Charlemagne's reign which are less often discussed because they do not fit well with the pleasing image of a wise, benevolent monarch in whose name religion and culture flourished.

Consider Charlemagne's war against the Saxons. This was a series of fierce conflicts that doggedly persisted from 772 - 804, with numerous treaties and truces that inevitably gave way to further battles. In the biography of Charlemagne, produced by the court official Einhard in about 830, the war is said to have been undertaken by Charlemagne to put an end to the incessant raiding and other misdeeds of Saxons on the borderlands of the Frankish kingdom.[5] Einhard would have us believe that this was a purely defensive war, but it is obvious from his account, that Charlemagne was determined to expand his empire by conquering the Saxons and converting them to Christianity. These are not separate issues for Charlemagne: he did not cease hostilities until the Saxons renounced their own religion and embraced Christianity. The refusal of the Saxons to abandon their ancestral traditions helps to explain the prolongation of the war for over thirty years.

Einhard observes that, "the war could have been brought to a more rapid conclusion, had it not been for the faithlessness of the Saxons": this 'faithlessness' was seen as the Saxons' continual refusal to fully accept Christianity and, in Einhard's phrase, "abandon their devil worship."[6] From Einhard's Christian-privileging perspective, the Saxons were stubborn, deceitful infidels, whose unchristian ways fully justified the use of massive force against them.

However, if we consider the situation from the point of view of the Pagan Saxons, a different picture emerges. From this perspective, the Franks, and especially their king Charles, were warrior-fanatics with a relentless desire to impose their religion. Whatever else might be said against the Saxons, there is no indication that they were trying to force their religion on the Franks. If we take seriously that the Saxons had their own religious traditions which they were trying to preserve from the Frankish onslaught, then their sustained refusal to accept a foreign religion being imposed on them by force, takes on a very different aspect from that suggested by Einhard. They were not stubborn or deceitful, but steadfastly pious and willing to give their lives to defend their faith.

Long before the onset of Charlemagne's campaigns against the Saxons, Christian missionaries had become active in the lands of the Saxons and other Germanic peoples.[7] When methods such as preaching and reasoning failed to convince Germanic Pagans to abandon their ancestral traditions, missionaries often resorted to more forceful methods. The Anglo-Saxon missionary Boniface for example, chopped down a sacred oak tree in the village of Geimar, in the region of Hessia, in order to demonstrate the superiority of the Christian god to the Pagan god associated with oak.[8] After this act of destruction, Boniface added insult to injury by confiscating the wood from the fallen sacred oak and using it to build Christian churches.

Such desecration and destruction of Pagan sacred sites and objects became an accepted missionary practice during this period.[9] It was with just such an act of religious aggression that Charlemagne inaugurated his hostilities against the Saxons. In 872, Charlemagne's army entered a Saxon town on the river Drimel and destroyed a sacred wooden pillar, known as the *Irminsul*. The Irminsul, apparently a decorated tree-trunk, was highly venerated in the religious observances of the Saxons as a representation of the world-tree.[10] Charlemagne's destruction of the world-tree proved to be an apt metaphor for his wholesale devastation of Saxon people, property, society and culture over the next thirty-two years. This attack on highly sacred sites and artefacts must have aroused powerful feelings of outrage amongst the Saxons and other Pagan peoples: not unlike the vociferous reactions generated by the September 11, 2001 attack on the World Trade Center in New York.

Christian sources such as saints' lives and missionary correspondence routinely claimed that such acts of destruction were highly successful in gaining converts to Christianity. They explained this supposed success with rather curious logic. In a letter to Boniface from the year 723, Daniel of Winchester observed:

> If the gods are all-powerful, beneficent and just, they not only reward their worshippers but punish those who reject them. If, then, they do this in temporal matters, how is it that they spare us Christians who are turning almost the whole earth away from their worship and overthrowing their idols?[11]

These missionaries obviously believed that their ability to destroy Pagan objects without incurring the wrath of Pagan deities proved the non-existence of these gods and by extension, the total absurdity of the religion. These authors never asked themselves whether the same might not apply to their own religion, that is, if the merits of Christian faith would be disproven by God's refusal to forcefully respond to the burning of a church or the cutting in half of a crucifix.

The same sources that boast of missionary successes through such acts of religious terrorism as the Irminsul destruction, cannot hide the massive retaliation by the Saxons and other peoples when their sacred traditions were threatened by Christian attacks. The Saxons repeatedly attacked and burned Christian churches, often carrying off their treasures in much the same way as Boniface had carted away the wood from the sacred oak at Geismar. In a letter to Pope Stephen III, Boniface apologizes for a delay in writing, explaining that he has been busy restoring thirty churches plundered and burned by Pagan rebels.[12] Above all, the fact that Charlemagne's destruction of the Irminsul ushered in thirty-odd years of warfare before the Saxons would surrender to Charlemagne and accept the religion of the Franks, implies that such actions were as likely to incite resistance as win converts.

Thirty-two years of war are bound to produce an abundance of bloodshed and death, but there is one particular action of Charlemagne's that stands out for its excessive cruelty. In 782, Charlemagne had, in one day, more than 4,000 Saxons beheaded for rebelling against Frankish rule and resuming the practice of their traditional Pagan religion after having previously signed a treaty agreeing to accept Christianity and Frankish domination. Such harsh measures did not end with the final surrender of the Saxons in 804. Charlemagne imposed stringent conditions of surrender upon the Saxons, prescribing capital punishment for a wide range of offenses, including many that were religious in nature.[13] Anyone who stole from a church, ate meat during the Christian fast of Lent, remained a Pagan and refused to undergo baptism, or engaged in a conspiracy of Pagans against Christians, was to receive the death penalty. At the same time, Saxons were required to provide labour, food and other support to churches and priests.

Modern historians of European religious history such as Kenneth Scott Latourette have not failed to register their regret at the massive loss of life and social devastation caused by Charlemagne's policies and methods, but they rarely raise the question of what right Charlemagne and his Christian comrades had to use military force to wipe out the religious life of a whole nation and compel conversion to a foreign religion. From the point of view of Christian privilege, such 'sins' are easily forgiven. As Latourette puts it, "However much the methods of Charlemagne may have been an innovation and a contradiction of the original spirit of Christianity, in the case of the Saxons they resulted in a permanent conversion."[14] Fletcher applies an ends-justifies-the-means argument, in that the sufferings of the non-Christians were justified by the triumph of Christianity: he writes, "It is well to remind ourselves ... that what was at issue was not the here and now but the eternal things: a God who could give salvation."[15]

Charlemagne's cruelty and intolerance in the war against the Saxons never detracted from his popular image as a wise and benevolent sovereign. His actions also appear to cause no concern to some people today who see Charlemagne as an attractive symbol of European unity. If we take the Pagan point of view however, Charlemagne appears to be the exemplar of religious intolerance, persecution and imperialism, the forefather not of European unity, but of some of the most problematic and shameful acts in European history. Charlemagne's war against the Saxons set the tone for the European Crusades and Inquisition, and paved the way for religious wars, persecutions and pogroms of the future.

What might have happened if Charlemagne had chosen a different path. What if he had pursued a policy of religious tolerance instead of religious persecution? What if he had offered the Saxons the option to join his empire without giving up their ancestral traditions? Thirty-two years of war could have been avoided, and a European civilization of tolerance and pluralism may have replaced one of intolerance and fanaticism. If Charlemagne had chosen a different path, perhaps he really would be an appropriate hero and symbol for our time.

2.   Revisiting the Vikings

If the popular view of Charlemagne has benefited from a rose-tinted treatment at the hands of Christian-privileging historians, then the seafaring Scandinavians of the 9th, 10th and 11th centuries, the Vikings, might be said to suffer from the reverse problem: their historical image is one of bloody, greedy, rapacious aggressors; products of a primitive culture and religion. This highly negative portrait, based largely on the writings of Medieval Christian authors, has been undergoing substantial revision in recent years, mainly due to the mounting body of archaeological research that suggests Vikings were builders and traders as well as destroyers and raiders. No one would deny that they were capable of great violence and savagery, but we can now see quite clearly that the Vikings were also a peaceful and productive people.

One of the reasons for the reputation attached to the Vikings, is that they obviously had little sense of public relations. In Medieval times any leader or group of people who wished to be loved and well-regarded needed to take great pains to gain the favour of the writers of authoritative historical records and propagators of public opinion. Viking leaders were very good at this within their own communities, heaping honours and treasures on poets and bards who literally sang their praises.[16] Icelandic literature contains many examples of such praise-poetry, celebrating the valiant careers of chieftains and kings from Viking times and earlier ages. Tapestry fragments in graves, suggests that decorative art probably served a similar function among elite classes. However, when the Vikings went abroad, they did not merely fail to flatter and bribe people in a position to influence their reputations, they raided, robbed and sometimes killed, thus motivating these opinion-makers and record-keepers to detail as dark a portrait of the Vikings as possible. That is to say, Medieval historical records were mainly written by Christian monks and priests, so when the Vikings repeatedly attacked and pillaged Christian monasteries and churches, the scribes ensured that they would be remembered as monsters, murderers and infidels.

For the Christian chroniclers, it was not only the Vikings' violence and greed that inspired their revulsion toward the Northmen, but the fact that the Vikings were non-Christians, worshipping gods and practicing traditions totally *other* to Christianity. From the Christian point of view, the Pagan Vikings not only behaved like devils, but worshipped them as well.

The Christian portrait of the savage, demonic Vikings is coherent and unified. It is however, one-sided. It only tells us of the Vikings aggressive behaviour in foreign lands, it does not give any account of Viking society or lifestyle in their native lands. In this way, the historical image of the Vikings is almost the opposite to that of Charlemagne and the Carolingian kingdom. Where Charlemagne's acts of cruelty and savagery toward the Saxons and other peoples were minimized and rationalized by situating them in the background of his more positive achievements in supporting church-based arts and culture in the Frankish kingdom, the Vikings' violence and destructiveness in raiding and attacking Christian lands was magnified by the absence of any information about other aspects of their culture.

From the Pagan point of view, we find reason to praise and celebrate the Vikings, not for their undeniable acts of savagery, but for their ingenuity, arts and literature, and above all, the way they defended their ancestral religious traditions against the rising tide of Christianization sweeping north towards Scandinavia. Their attacks on Christian institutions, usually seen as nothing more than missions of plunder, may be viewed as counterattacks against the aggressive growth of Christianity. This comes into sharper focus if we compare the chronology of Viking activities with important events in Christian expansion. The first Viking attack on a major Christian institution was the attack on the British monastery of Lindisfarne in 793, contemporary with the Frankish war against the Saxons, eleven years after Charlemagne's mass beheading of Saxon Pagans and some twenty one years after his attack on the Saxon temple containing the sacred oak pillar the Irminsul. Though Lindisfarne was not part of the Frankish kingdom, the Northmen were probably aware that many Christian missionaries came to the continent from Britain. An assault on a major British Christian site therefore, might have been thought of as a way of striking at the source of this anti-Pagan aggression. The fact that Lindisfarne was relatively unprotected and vulnerable undoubtedly added to its attractiveness as a target.

The motivations for Viking raids on churches and monasteries have been debated for many years, and the recent trend has been to emphasize the economic dimension, reasoning that the main motivation for attacking Christian sites could only have been to acquire the gold and other valuables contained in these houses of God.[17] By suggesting a possible religious dimension to Viking assaults on Christian institutions, I do not mean to dispute the obvious profit motive, but merely assert that there were very likely a number of different and overlapping motivations and purposes. As churches and monasteries were the repositories of great wealth as well as centres of religious and political authority, Viking raids on these sites no doubt enabled the simultaneous fulfilment of a wide range of objectives - military, political and religious, as well as economic. The same could be said of the Frankish assault on Pagan temples and sanctuaries in Saxony and elsewhere. Pagan sites often possessed wealth that Christian attackers would not hesitate to steal.

If we take the Vikings seriously, and not simply dismiss them as savage, rapacious brutes, I think we can view the various raiding and military activities of the Vikings as progressively large-scale and highly organized Pagan counterattacks against Christian, and particularly Frankish, expansion and imperialism. Just as the Franks went from small-scale attacks on Saxon border areas to large-scale conquest and colonization, so did the Vikings progress from hit-and-run raids on coastal sites like Lindisfarne in the late 8th century to mass invasion and colonization of England, Scotland, Ireland and other areas in the 9th century and beyond. It is to be noted that invading Vikings were often able to come to terms with local political authorities, but continued to devastate Christian institutions. For example, when the so-called 'Great Army' of Danish Vikings conquered the English kingdoms of East Anglia and Northumbria between 865 and 867, they quickly reached an agreement with the local people and their rulers, but brutally ravaged the Whitby monastery.[18] In such an instance, it would seem that the Vikings had a grudge against the Christians.

The hypothesis that Viking activities were a form of Pagan retaliation to Christian and Frankish expansion, is further supported in the cultural sphere. Between the 8th and 11th centuries, there was an impressive flowering of Pagan art and literature in Northern Europe, what we might describe as a Viking renaissance, roughly contemporary, and perhaps self-consciously competitive with the cultural resurgence sponsored by the court of Charlemagne, the so-called Carolingian renaissance. Many of the documents that we rely upon as source-materials for Nordic religion and mythology were first composed in this era, though our surviving texts are dated several hundred years later.[19] The theme of Valhalla, the afterlife paradise, ruled by Odin, the god of war, poetry and wisdom, where warriors feast and fight in preparation for a final, apocalyptic battle, is prominent on the famous runestone and picturestone memorials of the Baltic Sea island of Gotland from the 8th through the 11th centuries and in skaldic poetry of the 10th century. Contemporary royal tombs from Denmark and Norway, constructed on an impressive scale and luxuriously equipped with exquisitely carved and crafted objects, express a confident expectation of a joyful afterlife, a Pagan counterpoint to the proud monuments of the Christian faith being raised in the Frankish lands. The surrounding of these majestic Nordic royal tombs by lesser graves containing soldiers buried with weapons, riding gear, and even horses,[20] may echo the myth of Odin and his warriors dwelling together in the afterlife paradise of Valhalla.[21] One thing we can be sure of is that the Vikings did not view themselves as infidels or monsters. They had their own refined traditions, of which they were quite proud and all of which were threatened by the expansion of Christianity in Northern Europe.

When viewing the artistic, cultural and religious expressions of the Viking, we see a confident Pagan culture possessing great vitality, originality and refinement that was rooted in a rich and imaginative religious tradition. There is now an increasing appreciation for Viking artistry and culture, but this recognition was long delayed by the tendency to exclusively focus on the savagery of the Vikings. It is only with the deflation of the grand narrative of Christian supremacy, and in particular, the notion that European civilization is one and the same as European Christianity, that we are better able to appreciate the part that Viking and other Pagan cultures played in European history.

To close this discussion of the Vikings, let me again ask, as I did in regards to Charlemagne, *what if* ? What if the Vikings had not converted to Christianity? What effect would this have had on European history? From the Christian point of view, this would seem a nightmarish prospect. Viking religion is associated with idolatry and sacrifice, including human sacrifice. Such a perspective however, overlooks the important point that all religions change and develop over time. Just as Christianity has become more peaceful and tolerant over the centuries, refined and reformed through generation after generation of scholarship and theology, not to mention internal conflicts and upheavals, could not the same have happened, with the Pagan religion of the Vikings or other peoples, if they had been given the chance? We know that Hinduism, the majority religion of India, was once a religion of animal sacrifice with cattle as the preferred sacrificial victims. Over time and with the influence of new religious ideas, animal sacrifices fell out of favour and vegetarianism became established as a moral imperative, with cows seen as sacred animals to be protected. Could not a similar process of evolution and refinement have taken place with the Pagan religion of the Vikings? The answer cannot be known, because the Christianization of all Scandinavia closed the book on any further development of Norse Paganism.

Scattered pieces of information about Viking culture and society suggest that they were capable of accepting Christianity within their communities, as long as Christians did not undermine native Pagan traditions. Iceland for example, was settled by both Pagans and Christians, and the two religions coexisted in relative peace for more than a century. Archaeologists have found a number of graves in Iceland and elsewhere in Scandinavia that contain both hammer amulets, sacred to the Pagan god Thor, and Christian crucifixes, suggesting a syncretistic 'dual faith' in both Christianity and Norse Paganism.[22] The Eddas, sagas and other Old Icelandic literature likewise contain evidence of Christian-Pagan syncretism indicating that the Vikings were capable of combining Christianity with their own native traditions.[23]

In light of the evidence for Christian-Pagan syncretism, it would seem that the Vikings were not totally opposed to Christianity per se; rather, they attacked Christianity where it was perceived as part of a larger threat. Or to put it another way, they became aggressive against Christians in response to the aggression of Christians such as Charlemagne.

If Christian authorities had been willing to tolerate a more flexible kind of Christianity, a distinctive Nordic blend of Christianity and Paganism could have developed which might have served to bridge the two religious traditions and ameliorate conflicts between them. This was not to be. The powerful Christian authority structures of Medieval Europe were only interested in one kind of relationship with other forms of religion: the total destruction of these religions and the Christianization of all peoples, by force if necessary. Only now are we beginning to realise how much was lost as a result of those harsh policies of intolerance.

3. Conclusions

Today, the leaders of Europe and other highly developed regions have embraced the ideal of multiculturalism and pluralism, at least in rhetoric. This includes tolerance for other religions, not merely the various forms of Christianity that for so many centuries dominated the cultural life of Europe. I believe that if this 21st century experiment in pluralism and tolerance is to succeed, the history of Europe needs to be re-written to include the perspectives of non-Christian peoples of Europe's past, and to examine the processes by which ancient Pagan religions were wiped off the European map. If we accept the proposition that religious intolerance is a dangerous evil that has no place in the modern world, let us understand full well that it was just as dangerous, and just as evil, for the peoples of the past.

Notes

1. For lack of a better term, I will refer to these pre-Christian European religions as "Pagan" religions or as "Paganism."
2. The impressive but unfortunately biased studies of European Christianization of Kenneth Latourette 1938 and Richard Fletcher 1997 are prime examples of the ways in which unexamined assumptions of Christian superiority continue to influence scholarship in this area.
3. Bakhtin, 1981, 271-279.
4. On May 13, 1999, British Prime Minister Tony Blair was awarded the Charlemagne Prize, an annual award which has been granted since 1949 to political leaders and diplomats in recognition of their efforts to promote European unity. The prize, administered by the German city of Aachen, once one of the capitals of Charlemagne, has previously been granted to Winston Churchill, George Marshall, and Simone Weil, among others (*History Today* May 1, 1999). The British newsmagazine *The Economist* has a weekly feature on pan-European issues entitled *Charlemagne.*
5. Thorpe, 1971, 49-92.
6. Thorpe, 62.
7. Summarized with a distinctly pro-Christian bias in Sullivan, 1953, 705-740. For a more recent and balanced treatment see Cusack, 1998, 119-134.
8. Talbot, 1954, 43. See also Cusack, 123-127, and Latourette, 363.
9. Their ranks include Willibord, Sturmi, Liudger and Willehad. See Sullivan, 1953, 720.
10. Latourette, 389.

11. Emerton, 1940, 49-50.
12. Excerpted in Latourette, 373.
13. Boretius, 1897, 68-70. For translation, see Loyn and Percival 1975, 51-4. For discussion, see Karras, 1986, 552-572, and Fletcher, 214.
14. Latourette, 106.
15. Fletcher, 521.
16. Lonnroth, 1991, 3-10.
17. The viewpoint is summarized and critiqued in Lund, 1989, 45-60. See also Reuter, 1985, 75-94.
18. Roesdahl, 1991, 235-36.
19. Icelandic literature of the 12th and 13th centuries, composed some two to three centuries after the official conversion to Christianity, draws on oral traditions of Viking times and earlier periods, and provides crucial information about mythology and folklore, from a post-Christianization point of view. For discussion, see Aðalsteinsson, 1990, Dronke, 1996, and Kristjánsson, 1988.
20. Randsborg, 1980, 127.
21. Roesdahl, 1993, 131.
22. Fedotov, 1960, 3-10. For discussion of Thor hammer amulets, see Davidson, 1978, 113-127 and Roesdahl, 1993, 150.
23. Finnestad, 1990.

References

Aðalsteinnson, J. (1990), 'Old Norse Religion in the Sagas of Icelanders', *Gripla*, 7: 303-322.

The Avalon Project: Capitulary of Charlemagne Issued in the Year 802, at http://www.yale.edu/lawweb/avalon/medieval/capitula.htm.

Bakhtin, M. (1981), 'Discourse in the Novel' in *The Dialogic Imagination: Four Essays*, trans. by Caryl Emerson and Michael Holquist, Austin: University of Texas. 269-422.

Boretius, A. (ed.) (1897), *Capitularia regum Francorum. Monumenta Germaniae Historica Leges, sectio II*. Hanover, Germany: Impensis Bibliopolii Hahn.

Chamberlain, Russell. (1999), 'Blair Wins the Charlemagne Prize', *History Today* vol. 45, no. 5: 2.

Cusack, C.M. (1998), *The Rise of Christianity in Northern Europe 300-*

1000. London and New York: Cassell.

Davidson, H.R.E. (1978), 'Thor's Hammer', in: Davidson, *Patterns of Folklore*. Ipswich, UK and Totowa, NJ: DS Brewer and Littlefield, 113-127.

Dronke, U. (1996), *Myth and Fiction in Early Norse Lands*. Variorum Series. Brookfield, VT and Aldershot, UK: Ashgate Publishing.

Emerton, E. (trans.) (1940), *The Letters of Saint Boniface*. New York: Columbia University Press.

Fedotov, G. P. (1960), *The Russian Religious Mind: Kievan Christianity, The Tenth to the Thirteenth Centuries*. New York: Harper Torchbooks.

Finnestad, R. B. (1990), 'The Study of the Christianization of the Nordic Countries: Some Reflections', in: T. Ahlback (ed.) *Old Norse Religion and Finnish Cult-Place Names*. Abo, Finland: Donner Institute for Research in Religious and Cultural History, 265-272.

Fletcher, R. (1997), *The Barbarian Conversion: From Paganism to Christianity*. New York: Henry Holt.

Karras, R.M. (1986), 'Pagan Survivals and Syncretism in the Conversion of Saxony', *Catholic Historical Review* LXXII, 4: 552-572.

Kristjánsson, J. (1988), *Eddas and Sagas: Iceland's Medieval Literature*. trans. by Peter Foote. Reykjavík: Hið Íslenska Bókmenntafelag, 1988.

Latourette, K.S. (1938), *The Thousand Years of Uncertainty, A.D.500 – A.D.1500, A History of the Expansion of Christianity Volume II*. New York: Harper and Brothers.

Lonnroth, L. (1991), 'Sponsors, Writers and Readers of Early Norse Literature', in: Ross Samson (ed.) *Social Approaches to Viking Studies*. Glasgow: Cruithne Press, 3-10.

Loyn, R. and Pervical, J. (1975), *The Reign of Charlemagne: documents on Carolingian government and administration*. London: Edward Arnold.

Lund, N. (1989), 'Allies of God or Man? The Viking Expansion in a European Perspective', *Viator*. 20: 45-60.

Randsborg, K. (1980), *The Viking Age in Denmark*. London: Duckworth Press.

Reuter, T. (1885), 'Plunder and Tribute in the Carolingian Empire', *Transactions of the Royal Historical Society* vol. 5, no.3: 75-94.

Roesdahl, E. (1991), *The Vikings*. New York: Penguin.

Roesdahl, E. (1993), 'Pagan Beliefs, Christian Impact and Archaeology', in: A. Faulkes and R. Perkins (eds.) *Viking Revaluations*. London: Viking Society for Northern Research. 128-135.

Sullivan, R.E. (1953), 'The Carolingian Missionary and the Pagan', in *Speculum* vol. 28, no. 4 : 705-740.

Talbot, C.H. (trans. and ed.) (1954), *The Anglo-Saxon Missionaries in Germany*; *being the lives of SS. Willibrord, Boniface, Sturm, Leoba, and Libuin, together with the Hodoeporicon of St. Willibald and a selection from the correspondence of St. Boniface*. The Makers of Christendom. New York: Sheed and Ward. 43.

Thorpe, L. (trans.) (1971), *Einhard and Notker the Stammerer: Two Lives of Charlemagne*, Harmondsworth and Baltimore: Penguin Books.

Part II

Sexual Imagery: Locus of Pleasure, Pain, Censorship and Reclamation

The Female/Feline Morph: Myth, Media, Sex and the Bestial

Terrie Waddell

> *I often ask myself, just to see, who I am - and who I am (following) at the moment when, caught naked, in silence, by the gaze of an animal, for example the eyes of a cat, I have trouble, yes a bad time overcoming my embarrassment.*
>
> Jacques Derrida [1]

When morphing technology, animatronics, digital effects and Photoshop software developed as key special effects technologies in the late 80s-90s, anthropomorphic fantasy seemed irresistible. Contemporary cinema like *Babe, Pig in the City, Cats and Dogs, Men in Black II*, along with an overkill of screen and print advertising, were just more technically savvy examples of popular culture's fascination with human/animal hybrids. The desire to find union with animals, often thought to be abject and *other* to the superiority of human reason, has always been with us from screen character animation (c. 1912), cartooning/manga animal scrolls of the 12th century, a range of grotesque art dating back to Nero's Domus Aurea (Golden Palace), to the hunting and initiation images of the French and Spanish Palaeolithic grottos. This intermarriage however, is very one-sided - in our favour. Coming to terms with the animal *other* in a wider cultural context, often involves playing on notions of otherness by refashioning animals into quaint mutations of our female and male selves. Even when considering the most recent examples of human/beast composites it's a stretch to find gender neutrality in certain species, particularly when domestic pets are involved. As random and innocuous as the sexing of breeds may seem, this kind of gender assignment is far from arbitrary. Our anthropomorphic creations are grounded in an intricate coiling of history and mythology.

I've always been interested in the way in which cats have been associated with women when it comes to affecting a heightened sense of mystery, suspicion, duplicity, temptation, eroticism and evil. These associations might at first seem to be the reworked stuff of children's stories, but this female/cat baggage is much more deeply rooted in the archaic traditions of the 'Religious West'. As progressive as our culture might imagine itself, it still, almost unquestioningly, embraces ideologies that have long passed their used-by date. This becomes obvious when collectively acknowledged assumptions and associations that suture audiences to popular texts, are put under the microscope. The historical relationship between women and cats will be the prime focus of this chapter. By working through the sacred nature and subsequent corruption of this alliance, I hope to unravel the import of the contemporary female/feline combo.

1.   Hybrids of Antiquity

Before focusing on cats and their associations with women, it's useful to trace the obsessive way in which animals have been merged with humans. This creative preoccupation, which in ancient polytheistic religions was thought to honour and reconcile the power of the animal world, was revised with the onslaught of Christianity. The hybridizing of wo/man-beast largely became a way of conquering the irrational fear that surrounded the 'polluting' *other*. Perhaps the best example of this perversion of pagan icons is the demonizing of the Greek demi-god *Dionysos,* often pictured with the phallic man/beast silenoi and symbolised in the animal forms of goat, bull and snake. Fertility, change, danger, and sexuality were evoked through these 'genered' animals: the bull indicative of masculine strength and sexual potency, and the snake historically associated with fertility goddess cults of the early Minoan period. The familiar iconography of the Christian devil as a cloven-hoofed-half-man-half-beast (usually goat) was adapted from notions and images of the pagan *Pan/Dionysos* and stamped in the traditional and popular imagination as a craven figure to be feared as the evil shadow of the Christian god. Lucus Cranach's 16th century woodcut *Der Papstesel* (1523), is not only a grotesque image reminiscent of the ancient silenoi, but its breasts and lack of male genitals indicate a distinct femaleness. *Der Papstesel* and JakobRuoff's comparable image *The Devil Astaroth* (1539), are satirical mixes of all that transgressed. *Dionysos* was reinvented as a women/beast/devil and therefore reduced to a figure of ridicule.[2]

   The hybrid figures of myth - sphinx, siren, satyr, nixie, minotaur, mermaid, incubus, lamia, harpy, gorgan, centaur etc. – found their counterparts in the *grottesche* art movement of the late Middle Ages and Renaissance. The bizarre and excessive images of male and female forms interwoven with plants and animals intrinsic to the style, were adopted from frescos embellishing Nero's Domus Aurea.[3] The Roman form of *grotesque* art, dated at 100 BC, was copied from more ancient Asian cultures, which according to Geoffery Harpham, were influenced by pre historic cave paintings.[4] In Vitruvius' Treatise De Architectura (c. 27 BC) written during the rule of Emperor Augustus, the *grotto-esque* style was interpreted this way:

All those motifs which are based on reality, have now
been forsaken for an injudicious fashion. For
monstrosities are painted on the walls rather than clear
pictures of real things. Instead of columns, fluted stems
are painted; instead of gables (fastigis), panels with
curling leaves and volutes. Candelabra likewise support
painted edifices (aediculae). On their gables frail
flowers, on which random little figures sit, grow in
tendrils from their roots. And the slight stems actually
bear half-figures, some with human heads, others with
the heads of beasts.[5]

Fascination with the *grotesque* continued to influence Renaissance art and
architecture: Raphael (1483-1520), Giovanni Bellini (1430-1516),
Hieronymus Bosch (c. 1450-1516), Agostino Veneziano (1490-1540), Luca
Signorelli (1441-1523), Pieter Brueghel the Elder (1525-69) and Lucas van
Leyden (c.1489-1533) were among the more popular practitioners of the
style. The *grotesque* was used not only to decorate household items, posters,
art works, and private homes, but public and religious edifices as well.
Between 1499 and 1504 Signorelli was commissioned to paint the Cathedral
at Orvieto in the fashion; in 1502 Cardinal Todeschini Piccolomini
commissioned Pinituricchio to paint the ceiling of Sienna cathedral's library
in a similar manner; and in 1515 Raphael added ornamental *grotesqueries* to
the pillars of the papal loggias. These commissions indicate wide and
sanctioned appeal for the form.[6]

The *grotesque* not only captivated the public's imagination, but
according to Wolfgang Kayser, was also viewed as a dark and disturbing
realm of fantasy, "where the laws of statics, and proportion are no longer
valid. "[7] It stood in marked opposition to the structure of civilised Europe,
as something both alluring and sinister – the antithesis of reason and
culture. This was in part attributed to the interchange of human and animal
bodies - 'leaky', open, merging bodies - the kind of anatomy once ascribed
to women. To many Medieval and Renaissance thinkers, female
corporeality and the unbound, bestial and transgressive nature of the
grotesque were synonymous.

Attitudes toward animals during this period were also tainted
with superstition and anxiety. Foucault's writing on madness, which in the
Renaissance was crudely linked to notions of 'the beast', touches on the
irrational fear of being associated with animals and animality:

Western culture has not considered it evident that
animals participate in the plenitude of nature, in its

wisdom and its order: this idea was a late one and long remained on the surface of culture; perhaps it has not yet penetrated very deeply into the subterranean regions of the imagination. In fact, on close examination, it becomes evident that the animal belongs rather to an anti-nature, to a negativity that threatens order and by its frenzy endangers the positive wisdom of nature.[8]

The human/animal relationship continued to be problematic. Not only were animals associated with irrationality, but they also signified pollution, poverty and the 'untouchable' classes: as Peter Stallybrass and Allon White write of the 19th century, "the poor were interpreted as also transgressing the boundaries of the 'civilized' body and the boundaries which separated the human from the animal."[9] Much of the vitriol toward the bestial and hybridised human images has now vanished and some dignity has been restored, still ... echoes of previous discomforts remain. The woman/cat in popular culture for instance, gives us some insight into how we have appropriated past ideologies.

2.   Cat Gendering in Advertising, Film and Television

While cat/woman images aren't all-pervasive, contemporary play on the gendering of cats is a bit of a media fixation, especially in advertising ... so when a colleague tossed the latest print ad of the new 'X-type Jaguar' car across our staff table, I read this image of a naked woman digitally remade into a predatory jaguar, as a canny parody of the old assumptions linking women to the bestial - whether intended by the advertising creatives or not. The glossy 'X-Jag' poster-size spread was folded into four sections and inserted in *The Australian* newspaper, making this particular advertising launch difficult to miss. The poster is divided into images and structural information about the car, but because the product is pitched to a (very) financially independent female demographic, two of the largest shots are of women. One is a close up of the presumed consumer target, a young fresh faced, blue-eyed, blond, mid-late twenties business woman with the caption "The new Jag generation – the X-Type" running across the top of the image. The other is the more artistic long shot of the female/jaguar positioned on an upward sloping rock. The naked spotted figure, on all fours with back arched, strikes a stalking pose, as if concentrating on an invisible prey. The caption above the image is simply "Reborn" and below in smaller type "The art of performance, Jaguar" with an outline sketch of a leaping jaguar. The Australian arm of J Walter Thompson, the agency behind the account, presumably wanted audiences to 'get' that this model car is an evolved version of previous designs, revamped for a new female generation of upwardly mobile, sexy, independent, hungry, and ambitious Gen. X's. Qualities presumably signified by the 'big' cats.

Despite this shot being fairly representative of other media images were the female/cat mix combines enigmatic sexuality with predatory behaviour in order to fix a sense of power to the product under promotion, the jaguar was traditionally associated with male potency, particularly in Mayan art and ritual.[10] Men occasionally feature in glossy campaigns which intimate hybridization with cats, but in line with the Mexican theme, this matching, merging or morphing technique is used to accentuate ideals of strength and stamina. The latest Australian Slazenger sportswear spread is a typical example. In this print ad, run mainly in sporting magazines, close up images of men's faces, cropped at the forehead and chin so that the eyes, nose and/or mouth become the focus of the image, are positioned to the left of similar close-ups of panthers. Without direct digital enhancement a clear parallel is made between the panther and the face of an aggressive sportsman. While the current screen and print advertising for *Cadbury Schweppes* takes a different angle on male cats, by using digital syncing effects to humanize (and humourise) a male leopard into a poolside lothario, images of catwomen are far more sexual, sinister and shadowy: aggression is implied but rarely realised as physical strength or humour. The latency of menace is far more potent.

The recent Australian *Just Jeans* 'Whisker' campaign includes a television commercial where a young women walks to a birdcage and standing on a chair to reach the latch, takes the small bird, lovingly gazes at it, then stuffs it in her mouth. Even the close-up crotch shot of her jeans shows clear crease lines folding from the groin out so that they look like the outline of cat's whiskers. This of course helps fix the not so subtle link between the female genitals, often nick-named 'pussy', cats, cruelty and the notion of being vaginally 'devoured'. To have these very low cut, pubic enhancing, jeans is to be like the cat that swallowed the canary. Again cat-like women are cast as predators - hunters with a lack of conscience. Numerous advertisements revisit these old clichés. 'JAG' clothing and accessories for example often features the cool concentrated stare of a woman digitally remade into a leopard/ocelot, but my favourite image is from a promotional campaign for Guinness. It focuses, in tight close-up, on a woman's face. Her irises have been replaced by small pints of Guinness, making her large, directly gazing eyes, appear cat-like. She holds a pint of Guinness to her half open mouth and, in a not so subtle reference to the post ejaculation debris of fellatio, the head of froth from the glass sticks to, and drips from, her upper lip: a throw back to the death-swallowing vagina dentata of the cat.[11]

Kolotex's 'Voodoo winter hosiery' billboard, is one of the most controversial images to hit the Australian inner city - a far more racy play on hybridity than the previously mentioned advertisements. The image features a woman shot from the waist down, dressed in a tight fitting spotted mini dress, black leather gloves, red stockings and stiletto black leather boots cuffed with spotted patterning. She's holding a leash attached to the collars of two naked and totally clean shaven men crouching on hands and feet, so that they look like a pair of animals being taken for a walk. The image has clear bestial, dominatrix and sadomasochistic overtones. The woman, in her classical skin tight catsuitish gear, appears dominant, powerful and in her pointed heels, in a position to do some damage to her naked men if she was so inclined. Numerous complaints about the billboard were lodged with the Australian Advertising Standards Board, but they failed to take into account the ad's stinging play on gender and the gendering of certain animal species. Of particular interest were the objections toward humans, particularly men, being demeaned through their association with animals: "This is a moral issue that degrades human value and worth, it brings humans down to the level of animals" or "This kind of ultra feminism sends the totally wrong message to families where kids and young women think this is acceptable to treat men as 'pets' … it's emasculating and derogatory and heel grinding."[12] The ASB however, determined that the image, "represented a satirical comment on a patriarchal world" and therefore didn't contravene the Advertiser Code of Ethics.[13] While much 'shock' and 'distress' appeared to be caused through the dehumanizing of the male figures, little was made of the way in which the female image was more or less a response to previously constructed clichés of the relationship between women and cats.

Myth and popular culture have given us catwomen who tackle wickedness with seductive finesse. They arouse desire through their unattainably. They lure, hunt, scheme, and ensnare. Like Julia Kristeva's abject, they signify the irresistible pull to erasure.[14] They embody Freud's old play with sex and death. As Tom Gunning writes in relation to Jacques Tourneur's film *Cat People*, where the central character, Irena Dubrovna (Simone Simon), oscillates between human and panther incarnations: "In psychoanalysis, the figures of the fantastic, such as vampires or devils, [or cats] become interpreted as allegories of libidinal excess and conflict."[15] This notion of cats as signs of seduction and sexual permissiveness didn't escape Aristotle either, who thought that, "Female cats are naturally lecherous (*aphrodisiastikai*) and lure the males on to sexual intercourse, during which time they caterwaul."[16]

These common sex/death allusions to the cat as an independent, aloof and self-reliant seducer/hunter have been repeatedly personified in popular culture: the dominatrix suited catwomen Lee Meriwether, Eartha Kitt and Julie Newmar in the *Batman* television series, reinvented by Michelle Pfeiffer as Selina Kyle in *Batman Returns* and again to be made over by Ashley Judd in *Catwoman*; Nastassja Kinski as the panther obsessed Irena in Paul Schrader's remake of Tourneur's *Cat People*; Robert Wise and Gunther von Fritsch's *The Curse of the Cat People*; Madonna as the milk lapping erotic vamp in the video clip *Express Yourself* ; the artless cat with whom Pepi Le Pew becomes erotically intoxicated; and the cat morphing Professor Minerva McGonagall (Maggie Smith) in *Harry Potter And The Philosopher's Stone*, who, although sexually neutral, is still part of the 'Potter' phenomenon which Father Gabriele Amorth, the official exorcist of Rome, denounced as the work of Satan.[17]

Even leaving gender aside for a moment, it's difficult to find sympathetic animations of humanised felines. The film *Cats & Dogs* for example, exploits the cats-as-evil angle with arch villain Mr. Tinkles, the most recent in a pantheon of screen scoundrels including: Sylvester, Tom, Snowbell (in the film *Stuart Little*); evil Blofeld's lap cat in *From Russia With Love*; and Scott Carey's (Grant Williams) pet cat turned monster in *The Incredible Shrinking Man*. As journalist Christy Lemire writes, "Hollywood has its claws out for the kitties, consistently portraying them as scheming, devious and manipulative – and cats who talk are even worse."[18] This rationale oddly enough, extends to US Attorney Generals. John Ashcroft, a devout Pentecostalist, is claimed to believe that calico (multi-coloured) cats are signs of the devil, and in a no-so-unexpected extension of this logic, was also rumoured to have had the exposed breasts of Washington's Spirit of Justice statue covered with curtains.[19] Sex/women/cats, that old demonic triad, is still hard at work, gnawing at the sensibilities of puritans.

The contemporary examples mentioned above, are merely the postmodern upshot of more ancient histories and mythologies linking notions of evil and 'femaleness' to cats. With a keen intertextual eye, media savvy audiences are becoming increasingly deft at cross-referencing a vast array of multicultural images, narratives, chronicles, and artefacts in order to make sense of the popular. It is these skills that the creators of modern television, advertising and film rely on in order for their work to convey the intended meanings. I began by talking about how animal/human hybrids were traditionally imagined, I want now to trace more specifically, the links between women and cats, and through this reflection, illustrate how the very deep and intricate phases of this relationship have culminated in our present *reading* the female/feline.

3.   Divinities

Ancient Greek, Italian and Egyptian art and domestic artefacts - funerary pillars, tombstones, perfume bottles, vases, etc. - often associated and pictured cats with women. Female/feline names were common; Calpurnia 'Little Cat' or 'Kitten' (western empire); Cattula 'Little Cat' (Roman North Africa); Cattia Serena (Croatia).[20] Maenads were often distinguished by their familiarity with wild cats. In an ancient Greek racing cup, a maenad wearing a panther skin around her neck, holds a live panther by a hind leg (c. 480)[21]; perfume jars of the same period also image maenads in panther skins (c. 490 Athens, National Museum)[22]; and Picasso's Earthenware Vase of maenads in leopard skins (untitled, 1950), can be seen as a homage to these seductresses who were thought to lure 'respectable' women out of their homes and onto the streets during Dionysian festivals.

In the 22nd Egyptian Dynasty (945-715 BC), the capital Per-Bastet, or Tell Basta, was known for the 'House of the Goddess Bastet' or Bubastis to the Greeks. Although cat sacrifices took place, the animal was a sign of fertility and protection and was therefore sacred during this period. Killing a cat was a capital offence. According to Carol Andrews, in the early New Kingdom of Egypt, cat fetishes were a component of the insignia of female royalty: each wife of Tuthmosis III Pharaoh of the 18th Dynasty 1 (480 - 1426 BC): "once wore a bead bracelet with a spacer-bar surmounted by five reclining cats of gold, cornelian and composition. Gold-foil seated cats are also a component of the open-work amuletic collar of Queen Aahhotep."[23] During the Late Period Pakhet, the local goddess of Beni Hasan, had an entire graveyard of cat mummies devoted to her.[24]

Of all the Egyptian cat relics, Bastet is probably the most recognized idol. She functioned as the deity of motherhood and the hunt, and like Hermes and the Valkyries, acted as a psychopomp guiding the dead to the underworld. She was most often imaged as a cat-headed woman, but unlike other more ferocious female lion-headed goddesses, was generally connected with domesticity and fecundity:

> she carries a menyet collar with aegis-capped counterpoise and rattles a sistrum, both musical instruments connected with merry-making, but she nearly always has kittens near at hand as evidence of her fertility, occasionally carried in the round-bottomed basket which can hang over her arm.[25]

The sistrum, a type of rattle decorated with a small cat effigy, was commonly understood as a symbol of renewal and was also associated with Diana and Isis, who first introduced the principles of Bastet's cult to Western Europe: "In the Hellenistic Temple of Horus ay Edfu and inscription reads, 'Isis is the soul of Bastet,' that is, Isis can also become incarnate in a cat."[26] As Donald Engles writes:

> The cult of Isis and her sacred cat companion Bubastis was widespread and influential throughout the Roman Empire, both in the East and the West. Isis was originally an Egyptian divinity, whose cult was transformed when the Macedonians under Alexander the great conquered the region in 332 BC. At that time the native cult was suffused with Greek theological notions and artistic representations, The great temple of Isis and Sarapis at Alexandria, the Sarapeum, and its cult statues were some of the greatest religious monuments of the classical world.[27]

The cult of Bastet survived throughout the 1st millennium BC but continued via its fusion with the goddess worship of Artemis, Diana and Isis well into the Middle Ages.[28] The overthrow of pagan cults however, particularly those influenced by female deities, and the consequent condemnation of women in roles of authority, grew in intensity with the swelling power of Christianity. If the sects of Bastet (Egyptian), Isis (Greco-Egyptian), Diana (Italian) and Artimis (Greek) threatened the Christian West, then it's not surprising that cats, the signifiers of these matri-centered religions, were considered satanic.

4.   Demonisation of Female Deities

In the creation myth of Christian doctrine, man is given dominion over animals: "Let us make man in our image, in our likeness! Let them have authority over the fish of the sea and the birds of the heavens, over the cattle, over all the wild beasts and reptiles that crawl upon the earth!"[29] As Jacques Derrida writes, in relation to man's 'obligated' subjugation of all *other* creatures and of his power to 'name' those who existed before his inception:

> he has created man in his likeness so that man will subject, tame, dominate, train, or domesticate the animals born before him and assert his authority over them. God destines the animals to an experience of the power of man, in order to see the power of man in

> action, in order to see the power of man at work, in
> order to see man take power over all other living
> things.[30]

Derrida then returns to his cat, the pivot around which he explores the relationship between *otherness*, animals and the construction of identity:

> For so long now it is as if the cat had been recalling
> itself and recalling that, recalling me and reminding me
> of this awful tale of Genesis without breathing a word.
> Who was born first, before names? Which one saw the
> other come to this place so long ago? Who will have
> been the first occupant, and thus the master? Who the
> subject? Who has remained the despot, for so long
> now?[31]

I have included these thoughts, or as Derrida prefaces his argument "words of the heart", because it is from this shaping of masculine identity and sovereignty, born out of religious oppression, that we are able understand the enmity directed toward animals, the cat in particular, and as will be discussed later, women.

Catholicism spread throughout Europe by usurping pagan religions. While some traditions were maintained and incorporated into church practices, the essence of others, particularly female centred faiths that challenged the patriarchal monotheism of Christianity, were squashed. During the Middle Ages, pagan goddesses like the Germanic Perchta and the Roman Diana in particular, came to be associated with imaginary female collectives, 'sisterhoods' that bonded nocturnally with Diana, and performed subversive practices like the eating and reanimating of animals at the devil's behest.[32] This fabricated notion of sisterhoods was popularised in the *Canon Eposcopi*, a manual of regulations for bishops by the abbot Regino of Prüm (c. 892) who then processed the text for Archbishop Radbod of Trier.[33] The book influenced thinking in the later Middle Ages and was invaluable reference material for inquisitors in the witch hunting periods to follow. According to the text:

> It is also not to be omitted that some wicked women
> perverted by the devil, seduced by illusions and
> phantasms of demons, believe and profess themselves,
> in the hours of the night to ride upon certain beasts with
> Diana, the goddess of the pagans, and an innumerable
> multitude of women, and in the silence of the dead of

night to traverse great spaces of earth, and to obey her
commands as of their mistress, and to be summoned to
her service on certain nights.[34]

The cat, associated with Diana through her linkage to Isis and Bastet,
consequently became the signifier of these supposed Diana cults, and was
as a consequence, according to Engels, subject to, "suffering, cruelty and
virtual annihilation in many towns of continental Europe during the
Middle Ages ..."[35] Engels maintains that large groups of cats, particularly
black cats because of their sacred relationship to Isis also known as
'Queen of the Black Robe', were roasted alive in baskets: "Folk traditions
from later periods record that in many towns and cities, every single cat
was rounded up and tortured and burnt alive for local festivals. 'The cat,
who represented the Devil could never suffer enough'."[36] Walter Stephens
dates this relationship between cats and heretics back to the 12th and 13th
centuries, long before the hysteria of witchcraft reached its peak.[37] Pope
Gregory IX in his bull *Vox in Rama* (1233) wrote of black cats with erect
tails who morphed into pale men with black eyes, as incarnations of the
devil.[38] The obscene kiss of the black cat's anus, a ritual supposedly
practiced during clandestine gatherings of Cathars, was said by Alanus de
Insulis (12th century), to honour the devil – the allegation was, "a libel that
became commonplace, *Cathari* are so called from their worship of the
cattus, or cat."[39]
          Christian tyranny ensured that women were excluded from
political/public life and confined to the domestic sphere. Without a
collective voice, they were largely defined, accused and condemned by
men with whom they had little contact. Like the mute 'named' cat of
Derrida's writing, they were endowed, through religious fear and sexual
perversion/repression, with fantastical powers to incapacitate 'man' and
his god-given domination over beasts - the *others*, with whom women
came to be associated. Drawing on German artist Hans Baldung Grien's
images of naked women, witchcraft and the transgression of Eve,
Margeret Miles writes of Renaissance art and literature that, "the female
body at its most private and naked was presented as a symbol of specific
evil, not the general evil of the fall of 'man', but the carefully documented
evil of witchcraft."[40]
          The sexuality that we see in contemporary female/feline texts,
has a very specific history. The synonymous nature of death and sexual
allurement attached to cat/women is largely rooted in the delirium
surrounding the imagined practices of witches. The ancient worship of
cats and the ongoing domestic relationships that were maintained between
cats and their owners, was ruptured and debased as Christian doctrine took

hold of Europe. Any allusions to female power and autonomy were therefore brutally undermined. It seems odd that remnants of this irrational behaviour still filter through popular culture today. Although the independent nature of the cat as a species, (distinct from the popularly assumed loyalty of the dog for example), gives rise to personified versions of the cat as duplicitous and menacing, it is difficult to deny that much of Western history and the subsequent mythologies fostered by certain sweeps of faith, continues to inspire current interpretations of the cat-as-woman. These still recurring ways of seeing, can be traced to the nefarious goings on of 13th - 17th century demonologists.

5.   Cats, Devils, Witchcraft, Sex

In 1258 Pope Alexander IV ordered this inquisitors to hunt out witchcraft. The first mass witch trials of 1397-1406 took place at Boltinger in Swiss Lucerne and later in Valais and the Dauphiné in 1428.[41] Pope Innocent VIII's bull *Summuis desiderantes affectibus* of 1484, allowed inquisitors and ecclesiastical judges to eradicate sorcery: this edict has often been cited as the primary cause of much suffering for those accused of witchcraft in the 15th to 17th centuries. Two years later in Strasbourg, Heinrich Institoris published his *Hammer of Witches* (*Malleus Melficarum*) - required reading for 16th century demonologists.

The association of witchcraft with animals considered to manifest evil - asses, goats, rats, cats, crows, bats, bulls, toads etc. - continued throughout the witch hunts. Of all the creatures imagined to be the familiars and conduits for evil spirits, cats were probably the most maligned in terms of the fantasies woven around them and the physical abuse they endured. When Agnes Waterhouse, one the first executed for witchcraft in England, confessed in 1566 to keeping a cat named 'Satan' as her familiar, stories of the demonic nature of cats were already well and truly in circulation.[42] As early as 1427 Saint Bernardo of Siena revealed that he indicted a witch for murdering her child and thirty others, by using a emollient to affect the appearance of a cat, and in 1440, "the physician Antonio Guaineri recorded that 'our common people call [witches] *strigae* or *zobianae*, and say that they often assume the shape of cats'."[43] Strigae were thought of as night vampires who drank the blood of humans. A version of this type of supernatural being became known as a witch-cat, a creature that attacked infants and drank their blood. But because, so it was theorised that these creatures were able to instantly heal the puncture marks/wounds they would have had to have made in the child's flesh, they always escaped detection – like the best conspiracy theories, there's a loop-hole to compensate for lack of evidence. Stephens posits that the high incidence of infant death during the Middle Ages and the Renaissance, contributed to the folktales and supposed sightings of witch-cats, cats, and witches who preyed on young children: "If blood was ever found near babies, their death was obviously caused by demonic witch-cats even if no bite or scratch marks can be found."[44]

Chief Justice Henri Boguet (1550-1619) in his psychotically brutal manual for demonologists, *An Examen of Witches,* raves in excruciating detail about how to identify and torture witches and their accomplices; male, female, children, adolescents and familiars, who, according to Bouget's sources, were witches in disguise :

> Others have been changed into cats. In our own town one named Charcot of the bailiwick of Gez was attacked by night in a wood by a number of cats; but when he made the sign of the Cross they all vanished ... The Inquisitors also tell that in their time there were seen three large cats near the town of Strasbourg, which afterwards resumed the shape of women.[45]

This notion of shape-shifting also filtered through folk tales that described how abused cats then reappeared as women with 'tell-tale' signs of their beatings. In 1608 Francesco Guazzo described how a witch, after changing into the form of a cat in order to attack a child, was chased and battered until it fled through the window: Guazzo alleges claims that the cat then reappeared as a woman, "with a bruised and broken body".[46] Yet despite the anecdotes and claims that women and the devil transfigured themselves, it was also widely thought amongst Catholic demonologists (and Boguet himself) that these transformations were cunning illusions, not actual physical shifts from human to beast. This position was adopted in respect of the Canon *Eposcopi,* which held that only god could refashion the human body into an animal. Such convictions naturally demeaned pagan traditions where goddess like Diana and Circe were endowed with the power to change men into dogs and swine. The *Malleus Melficarum's* contention that witch-cats could steal penises, was also cited as evidence to support just how completely demons were able to distort human perception.[47] The phallus, biologically and as a signifier of masculine power, was not actually severed or threatened, but *thought* to be due to sorcery. This fear of genital mutilation, of being 'womanlike', can be understood as yet another means of marking out women as threats to the established order.

The witch-hunting period also associated cats and women with the extremes of sexual indulgence and perversion. Bestiality was thought to be akin to copulating with the devil. It was therefore believed that witches adopted this practice in a ritualistic fashion during the imagined gatherings known in the mid-15th century as 'sabbat'. Boguet of course, encouraged such delusions and wrote in detail of these kinds of activities in his *Examen*. This thinking was further supported by the ink etchings and woodcuts of Baldung Grien, renown for his imagery of witches during the height of the post-*Malleus* frenzy. Baldung's obsession with the madonna/whore dichotomy marked his career: he fantasized of the sexualised woman as an intimidating presence that threatened to overwhelm male authority, and imaged her as a naked version of either Eve or 'the witch'. He mainly drew witches as sexually active collectives of young and aged women, their large and/or wrinkled bodies writhing on one another while their familiars sat close by. In three of his most famous works all titled *Witches' Sabbath* - the woodcut (1510), pen on green tinted paper (1514) and pen on re-brown tinted paper (1514) - a large cat is curled up in the foreground. In the first image the cat is sitting back to back with the central witch who stirs the cauldron, while in the second and third images, the cat howls in accompaniment to the orgiastic play of the coven. The inclusion of cats amid these naked figures gives the impression of a collusive woman/beast relationship: the cat and the witch are physically separate, yet inseparable versions of a presumed corrupt, evil and polluting 'animalistic depravity'.

This belief in the leaky woman/beast margins was further intensified by the assumption that unusual raised marks or moles were often found on the bodies of witches. In a bizarre twist of logic, these blemishes, supposedly located on erogenous bodily zones, were thought to be nipples from which cats and other familiars suckled blood.[48] One may argue that the female body was enough of a 'leaky vessel' with its predisposition for menstruation, lactation and all the fluids of childbirth, but the disrespect for bodily boundaries signified through the witch's bleeding teats, her fusion with animals, and her sexual promiscuity, posed an irreconcilable threat to the Christian ideal of the contained body - clean, proper and unsullied by signs of abjection (blood, puss, excrement, death, decay etc.). These imagined transgressions were of course rabid fantasies, based on fear, ignorance and religious/sexual pathologies licensed by fanatics like Boguet.

6.   Women as Beast

Aside from the direct linkage of women with pagan cults, cats and later witchcraft, the Middle Ages and Renaissance (as mentioned earlier) were more generally periods when human separation from, and superiority to, plants, animals and the cosmos was supported by Genesis, where man (before woman) was created by a *male* god and privileged with domination over the natural world: 12th century Bishops, Marbode of Rennes, Hildebert of Lavardin, and Geoffroy of Vendome; Thomas Aquinas and Gilbert of Tournai (13th century); and Alvaro Pelayo and Gilles Bellemere (14th century), with their varying puritanical philosophies of reason used women as scapegoats - the intolerable *other* to define themselves against.[49] Miles' study of the female body in the Christian West, documents how femaleness was linked to animality and the intensity with which women were restrained from any form of public display. Those who transgressed the church's moral codes by expressing sexuality and desire were persecuted. This connection between women, sex and the bestial has also been popularised by writers and physicians of the 16th century who likened the uterus to, "a hungry animal; when not amply fed by sexual intercourse or reproduction, it was likely to wander about her body, overpowering her speech and senses."[50]

The perverse reasoning that linked women and animals, continued into and beyond the Enlightenment. When Europeans first settled in Australia, convict women's bodies, particularly prostitutes, signified social chaos and pollution: Joy Damousi writes that, "In these understandings of convict women, the bodily boundaries of animal and human were blurred and identified as a source of disorder."[51] A lieutenant colonel Godfrey Charles Mundy's visit in 1851 to a female prison in Tasmania, attests to this accepted fixing of women with the bestial. Here he offers his impressions of a young convict girl:

> when she purred loudest I should have been most afraid of her claws! ... the turkey informed me that this was one of the most refractory and unmanageable characters in the prison. That said beauty is a sad distorter of man's perceptions! Justice ought to be doubly blindfolded when dealing with her ... the pang of pity that shot across my heart when that pretty prisoner was shut again from the light of day, might have found no place there had she been as ugly as the sins that had brought her into trouble.[52]

Not only were female prostitutes and criminals associated with animals, but the slang word *scrubber*, now used to demean women known or assumed to be overtly sexual, can be etymologically traced to early Australian settlement. Borrowed from the English to describe one who forages, *scrubber* was incorporated into the Australian vernacular in the 1850s as a way of describing feral/unbranded farm stock or brumbies (wild horses) who mate randomly. This connection between undomesticated women and animals, that old Medieval/Renaissance initiative, remains a perverse point of connection between the old world and the new, that served to abject women from public positions of authority and political activism.

The notion that intellectual reason distinguishes humans from other life forms, and that it is considered an insult to smudge the margins or draw associations between women/men and animals, is still a commonly accepted prejudice. Take for instance one of the public responses to the Voodoo hosiery billboard mentioned earlier, where the imaging of men as dogs was thought to "bring humans down to the level of animals." Reason and containment are still valued over excess, instinct and emotion. The dichotomy is most clearly marked through our labelling of male and female genitalia, pussy and cock - sites of impulse, sensation, ecstasy and rebirth. These often publicly censored terms signify our 'base' or 'lower' urges - ongoing sources of pleasure, guilt, shame and punishment. Sex with all its irrational mastery over us, bonds us most closely with animals. It is an inescapable drive that although repressed to varying degrees throughout history, manages to find an outlet, no matter how pathological. Women's bodies which disclose sexual activity through pregnancy, have, since Eve's fall, been used to signify the way in which desire frustrates reason. This notion *of otherness* between men and women / human and animal, sets up a sharp and often cruel dualism that unfortunately still glues the framework of much contemporary popular culture and political thinking.

7.   Conclusion

How we experience female/animal images today varies according to the way in which we deconstruct these media texts in order to mine 'meaning'. Semiotic analysis alone robs our modern images of depth - it's simply naive to ignore the a-temporal nature of myth, clashing political doctrines and religious traditions that continue to inform our print and screen fictions. While the technologies of information transmission continue to develop, allowing us to experience imagery in a variety of forms, the essence of these 'messages' and the ideologies they support, can be traced to our earliest systems of communication. The creative teams behind advertising, print media, television and film, often either directly transplant or dissect and repaste elements of our lived and fabricated past in order to tap into the postmodern aesthetic that we now take for granted.

From gods who either physically morph into animals or are represented as human/animal hybrids, to Medieval woman-as-beast dogma, our 'X-type Jag' or 'Voodoo hosiery' woman (as a representative image) not only manifests the power of a deity, but also the baggage of the irrational, seductive *other*. The contemporary female/feline morph, in line with her predecessors, confronts audiences with a mixed bag of gender ideologies. By examining the import of the cat/woman and the beliefs that our culture still nurtures in relation to the way she is imagined, we are able to see ourselves in a broader context and in so doing question our attachment to the archaic vestiges of certain religious beliefs.

I'd like to finish where I began, with Derrida. The following question sums up much of my thinking throughout this chapter, for he embraces notions of *otherness* while acknowledging the interconnection between that *other* and ourselves, when he asks, "But cannot this cat also be, deep within her eyes, my primary mirror?"[53]

Notes

1. Derrida, 2002, 372.
2. *Der Papstesel, Lucas Cranach,* in Harpham, 1982 and *An illustration of The Devil Astaroth,* by JakobRuoff in Barry, 1966, 260.
3. Excavated from ancient Roman ruins in 1480 AD. Harpham, 1982, 23
4. Harpham, xi.
5. Thompson, 1982, v.
6. Kayser, 1981, 20-1.
7. Ibid., 21. This is contested by Mikhail Bakhtin (1984) who viewed the grotesque as intrinsic to the liberating, celebratory and 'socialist' principal of carnival.
8. Foucault, 1965, 77.
9. Stallybrass, 1986, 132. Also see Douglas, 1984, 113.
10. Coe, 1972, 10.
11. For more on 'vagina dentata' myths and popular media imagery see Creed, 1993. Also refer to Kristeva, 1982 for her reading of 'the abject'.
12. Wilson, 2002, www.
13. Ibid.
14. Catwoman figures in horror often classify as forms of what Creed calls, 'the monstrous feminine'. Creed, 83.
15. Gunning, 1988, 32.
16. Citied in Engles, 1999, 74.
17. Patterson, 2002, 18.
18. Lemire, 2001, L04.
19. Dowd, 2002, 27.
20. Engels, 99 & 105.
21. Lissarrague, 1994, 22-23.

22. Ibid., 227-9.
23. Andrews, 1994, 33.
24. Ibid., 34.
25. Ibid., 32.
26. Engels, 35.
27. Ibid., 115.
28. Ibid., 30-31.
29. Gen. 1:26-28; trans Chouraqui, in Derrida, 384.
30. Derrida, 386.
31. Ibid., 387.
32. Sallmann, 1993, 453-4.
33. Russell, 1972, 76.
34. Cited in Ibid.
35. Engels, 77.
36. Ibid., 159 also see pp.132-4 regarding the black cat's relationship to Isis.
37. Stephens, 2001, 281.
38. Russell, 161.
39. Stephens, 281.
40. Miles, 1991,127.
41. Sallmann, 446.
42. Rosen, 1991, 72-82.
43. Stephens, 285.
44. Ibid., 286.
45. Bouget, 1903, 142.
46. The incident is dated approx. 1576, as reported by another Italian demonologist in that year. Guazzo, 1988, 51.
47. Stephens, 291-302.
48. Karlsen, 1987, 137.
49. Dalarun, 1992, 15-41.
50. Zemon Davis, 1975, 124.
51. Damousi, 1997, 38.
52. Ibid., 50-51.
53. Derrida, 418.

References

Andrews, C. (1994), *Amulets of Ancient Egypt.* London: British Museum Press.

Arnold, J. (director). (1957), *The Incredible Shrinking Man.* [film]. Universal International Pictures. USA.

Bakhtin, M. (1984), *Rabelais and his World* Iswolsky (trans) (1965) Bloomington: Indiana University Press.

Barry, G., J. Bronowski, J. Fisher, J. Huxley. (eds) (1966),*The Arts: Man's Creative Imagination* London: Aldos Books.

Boguet, H. (1929), *An examen of witches.* Rev. M. Summers (ed). London: J. Rodker.

Burton, T. (director). (1992), *Batman Returns.* [film]. PolyGram Pictures and Warner Bros. UK and USA.

Coe, M. D. (1972), 'Olmec Jaguars and Olmec Kings', in: E. P. Benson (ed.) *The Cult of the Feline: A Conference in Pre-Columbian Iconography,* Washington D.C: Dumbarton Oaks Research Library and Collections, 1-13.

Columbus, C. (director). (2001), *Harry Potter And The Philosopher's Stone.* [film]. 1492 Pictures, Heyday Films, Warner Bros. UK.

Creed, B. (1993), *The monstrous Feminine, Film feminism, psychoanalysis*, London: Routledge.

Dalarun, J. (1992). 'The Clerical Gaze', in: C. KlapischZuber. (ed). *A History of Women in the West: Vol. Two, Silences of the Middle Ages.* Massachusetts: The Belknap Press of Harvard University Press.

Damousi, J., (1997). *Depraved and Disorderly: Female Convicts, Sexuality and Gender in Colonial Australia.* Cambridge: Cambridge University Press.

Derrida, J. (2002), 'The Animal That Therefore I am (More to Follow)'. David Wills (trans). *Critical Inquiry*, 28:2. 369-419.

Dowd, M. (2002), 'A Blue Burka for Justice', *New York Times*, 30 January. 27.

Douglas, M. (1984), *Purity and Danger: An Analysis of the Concepts of Pollution and Taboo.* ARK: London.

Dozier, W. (executive producer). (1966-68), *Batman.* [television series]. 20th Century-Fox. USA.

Engels, D. (1999), *Classical Cats: The Rise and Fall of the Sacred Cat.* London: Routledge.

Fincher, D. (director). (1989), *Express Yourself.* [video clip]. USA.

Foucault, M. (1988), *Madness and Civilization: A history of Insanity in the Age of Reason.* Trans. Richard Howard. New York: Random House.

Guazzo, F.M. (1988), *Compendium Maleficarum*, in: M. Summers, M. (ed). Ashwin, E.A. (trans). New York: Dover. pp..

Gunning, T. (1988), ' "Like Unto a Leopard" Figurative discourse in Cat People (1942) and Todoro's The Fantastic'.*Wide Angle*, 10:3. 30-39.

Guterman, L. (director). (2001), *Cats and Dogs.* [film]. NPV Entertainment, Village Roadshow Productions, Warner Bros., Zide-Perry Productions. USA and Australia.

Harpham, G., (1982), *On the Grotesque: Strategies of Contradiction in Art and Literature.* New Jersey: Princeton University Press.

Karlsen, C. F. (1987), *The Devil in the Shape of a Woman: Witchcraft in colonial New England.* New York: W.W.Norton and Company.

Kayser, W. (1981), *The Grotesque in Art and Literature.* U. Weisstein. (trans) (1957). New York: Columbia University Press.

Kristeva, J. (1982), *The Powers of Horror*, L. S. Roudiez (trans) New York: Columbia University Press.

Lemire, C. (2001), 'Cats aren't top dogs at the movies'. *The Advertiser.* 13 September. L04.

Lissarrague, F. (1994), 'Figures of Women', in: P. Schmitt Pantel. (ed). *A History of Women: From Ancient Goddesses to Christian Saints,* Massachusetts: Harvard University Press.

Miles, M. (1991), *Carnal Knowing: Female Nakedness and Religious Meaning in the Christian West.* New York: Vintage.

Miller, G. (director). (1998), *Pig in the City.* [film]. Kennedy Miller Productions. Australia and USA

Minkoff, R. (director). (1999), *Stuart Little*. [film]. Columbia Pictures Corporation, Franklin/Waterman Productions and Global Medien KG. USA and Germany

Noonan, C. (director). (1995), *Babe*. [film]. Kennedy Miller Productions and Universal Pictures. Australia and USA.

Patterson, B. (2002), 'Exorcist sees Devil in Harry'. *Herald-Sun*. 6 January. 18.

Pitof (director). (2003), *Catwoman*. [film]. Warner Bros. USA

Rosen, B. (ed) (1991), *Witchcraft in England, 1558-1618*. Massachusetts: University of Massachusetts Press

Russell, J. (1972), *Witchcraft in the Middle Ages*. London: Cornell University Press.

Sallmann, J. (1993), 'Witches', in: N. Zemon Davis and Arlette Farge (eds). *A History of Women: Renaissance and Enlightenment Paradoxes*. Massachusetts: Harvard University Press. 444-457.

Schrader, P (director). (1982), *Cat People*. [film]. RKO Pictures and Universal Pictures. USA.

Sonnenfeld, B (director). (2002), *Men in Black II*. [film]. Amblin Entertainment, Columbia Pictures Corporation and MacDonald-Parkes. USA.

Stallybrass, P. and A. White. (1986), *The Politics and Poetics of Transgression*. London: Methuen.

Stephens, W. (2002), *Demon Lovers: Witchcraft, Sex and the crisis of Belief*. Chicago: The University of Chicago Press.

Thompson, J. (1982), *Monty Python: Complete and Utter Theory of the Grotesque*. London: BFI Publishing.

Tourneur, J. (director). (1942), *Cat People*. [film]. RKO Radio Pictures Inc. USA.

Wilson, P. (2 July, 2002), 'Strategic disempowerment'. *Wilson's Almanac*.

http://www.wilsonsalmanac.com/voodoo.html

Wise, R. and G. von Fritsch (directors). (1944), *The Curse of the Cat People*. [film]. RKO Radio Pictures Inc. USA.

Zemon Davis, N. (1975), *Society and Culture in Early Modern France*, Stanford, Ca: Stanford University Press.

Young, T. (director). (1963), *From Russia With Love*. [film]. Danjaq Productions and Eon Productions Ltd. UK.

Bad Sex:
Second-Wave Feminism and
Pornography's Golden Age

Loren Glass

The opening of Gerald Damiano's hard-core film *Deep Throat* at New York's World Theater on June, 1972 marks a turning point in American cultural history. Over six thousand people went to see it in the first week. Mainstream reviewers praised it. Its New York success sparked a nationwide run, giving Middle America a strong dose of coastal cosmopolitan culture. The film, which originally cost only $25,000 US. to make, eventually grossed over $25,000,000 making it one of the most profitable films of all time. It remains one of the top-selling hard-core video rentals. The unexpected success of *Deep Throat* seemed to signal the apogee of America's sexual revolution, heralding a new age of frank and uninhibited public engagement with intimate issues previously suppressed by Puritanism and prudery. Its focus on one woman's quest for sexual satisfaction additionally seemed to indicate that the double standard was finally being overturned; female pleasure was finally being acknowledged in the public sphere.

Within six months however, the film was banned in New York, and indeed in many other localities across the country. Later that year the Supreme Court, now headed by Nixon appointee Warren Burger, had ruled on the case of *Miller v. California*, altering the legal definition of obscenity, which had been narrowed down to almost nil by the famously liberal Warren Court. The ruling in *Miller v. California* determined that local, as opposed to national, community standards could be used to define obscenity. It also replaced the "utterly without redeeming social value" clause with "lacks serious literary, artistic, political, or scientific value."[1] The brief 'Golden Age of Pornography' was over, but the century-long battle over the definition and regulation of porn in America was not. In fact the battle lines had received new energy and emphasis from feminism's equally brief second wave, which took the sex industry as one of its foes in the fight for social, and sexual, equality. In this chapter, I will interrogate the complex coincidence of porn's golden age and feminism's second wave. Both emerged at the close of the 1960s, enjoyed a brief period in the media spotlight, and essentially ended by the mid-70s. The consequences of and relationship between both phenomena remains the subject of debate.[2]

The engagement between pornography and feminism generated some peculiar political allegiances: radical feminism partnered with right-wing fundamentalism in the effort to suppress porn, while academic feminists allied with porn industry profiteers in the effort to protect it. *Deep Throat,* as one of the most well-known hard-core films of the era, figured prominently in this battle. The female lead, Linda Lovelace, played something of a starring role, particularly after she went public with accounts of abuse and mistreatment by her manager/husband before, during, and after the making of the film. Having started out as the mouthpiece for the libertarian, hedonistic ethos at the extreme end of the anti-censorship camp, she ended up being the exemplary victim for the anti-pornography activists.

Linda Lovelace, as the woman who once bore her name readily admits, was a fictitious person, a placeholder for the powerful fantasies and anxieties at work in the debate over pornography. As such, she can be analyzed as a public subject, embodying and condensing the contradictory attitudes about gender and sexuality that emerged in the wake of feminism and the sexual revolution.[3] Her invention and transformation in the public sphere provides an illuminating dialectical link between feminism and pornography in the 70s and 80s. That link, I hope to argue, is the culture of celebrity, the process whereby a public subjectivity is generated through the sheer process of its circulation as a commodity in the mass-mediated public sphere.

Scholars of fame in America agree that the post-WWII era witnessed a dramatic expansion of celebrity discourses and practices into political realms that previously, at least in theory, bracketed personal concerns.[4] President John F. Kennedy is usually positioned as the central figure in this regard; his telegenic good looks and sexual allure brought movie star power to the White House. His glamorous wife, storybook family, and high-society social life were tightly integrated into his political image. Later, the tabloid exposure of his many affairs would only enhance his celebrity image, and affirm the interpenetration of public and private life that such images embody.

Both the sexual revolution and feminism were implicated in this expansion of the culture of celebrity, insofar as both emphasized bringing private issues into public discussion. During the 60s, censorship in both literature and film was relaxed almost to the point of non-existence, enabling the enormous popularity of unprecedentedly explicit works such as *Portnoy's Complaint* and *Midnight Cowboy.* Correlatively, feminism's insistence that 'the personal is political' implicated these explicit representations in a critique of American gender relations. Celebrities like Linda Lovelace, I will argue, begin to emerge as symptoms of this collapsing divide between public and private realms.

These new celebrities tend to indicate the contradictions in, and the limits of, the political transformations envisioned during the height of feminism and the sexual revolution. In particular, I hope to show how the celebrity discourses that emerged in the wake of feminism and the sexual revolution reveal how the interpenetration of public and private, rather than mitigating or eliminating conventional gender roles, tend to exaggerate them by enhancing the public focus on genital sexual difference. Although one might argue that celebrities prove the performative nature of gender identity, there is a strong counter current in which celebrities essentialize such identities by collapsing gender into sex.

The figure of Linda Lovelace illustrates this process whereby the imaginary fantasy of public performance and the empirical reality of private experience become crucially confused. Indeed, the evidentiary function of her body and her words reveals how both pornography and celebrity foreground the link between public and private as, ultimately, epistemological. For those who defend porn, she is proof of female pleasure; for those who condemn it, she is proof of female victimization. This evidentiary function indicates how porn focalizes our desire for sexual knowledge. It is the epistemological ground of American fantasies about sexuality and gender relations, proving the ultimate reality of both the pleasure and the pain that these fantasies provoke.[5] That Linda Lovelace could prove both things indicates that contemporary celebrity and mainstream pornography operate within congruent fields, where the individual body in the public sphere validates our deepest desires and anxieties about the nature of sex under late capitalism. The shift in her evidentiary function from female pleasure in the early 70s to female victimization in the late 70s and early 80s provides a convenient emplotment for the complex engagement between feminism and pornography in the wake of the 60s sexual revolution.

1.   Legitimating Linda

This emplotment can best be unpacked through a reading of the series of autobiographical books that appeared in her name in the decade after the opening of *Deep Throat*. The first was *Inside Linda Lovelace*, a combination intimate exposé and sex manual published in 1973 to capitalize on the unexpected popularity of *Deep Throat*. On the flyleaf appears a signed prefatorial remark that reads (in part): "This is My Story. I lived it. I wrote it ... I'm doing exactly what I want to do, how I want to do it, when I want to do it, and with whom I want to do it."[6] Furthermore, she avers, "If I put something in writing it has to be the truth, and I mean the full truth."[7] The narrative that follows plots its subject's autobiography around the development of a hyperbolic hedonism. As a girl she was, "an incorrigible masturbator"[8]; she got so good that she can now think herself "to orgasm."[9] She claims, "My God is now sex. Without sex, I'd die. Sex is everything."[10] She feels that, "what goes on between kids is great. The same for adults, and it makes no difference to me personally if adults make it with kids, boys with boys, Grandpas with granddaughters or whatever."[11] She also bills herself as a new age sex expert, advising techniques of meditation and self-hypnosis to improve performance and enjoyment. *Inside Linda Lovelace* then, provides its subject with both agency and expertise, but only in the service of legitimating the 'truth' of her sexual pleasure.

Inside Linda Lovelace is dedicated to her manager/husband "Chuck Traynor - the creator", who Lovelace would later claim wrote the text for her. She then dictated the text into a tape recorder for Pinnacle Books, to whom it is copyrighted, with special thanks to "Mr. Douglas Warran for his editorial assistance." Pinnacle would also publish Lovelace's next book, *The Intimate Diary of Linda Lovelace* (1974), in which she would declare her independence from the abusive Traynor, thereby giving her story a further feminist flavour. Having finally escaped from the man who beat and imprisoned her, Lovelace proclaimed, "Nobody will put ideas in my head or words in my mouth again. What I say and what I do is strictly me. I am nobody's piece of property. I am my own person."[12] And again she affirms: "What I do is only the truth."[13] *The Intimate Diary* attempts to ballast the hedonistic ethos of the earlier book by providing a broader public - and quasi-feminist - frame for its subject's agency and independence. In this book Linda Lovelace goes out into the world, hobnobbing with celebrities and struggling with the law. Nevertheless, this text is also copyrighted to Pinnacle and appears "as told to" a man named Carl Wallin.

Indeed, it is impossible to determine how much of these two texts were written by the woman who bore the name in the title. In her two later confessional texts - *Ordeal* (1980) and *Out of Bondage* (1986) - Lovelace completely disavows the identity and agency claimed by the first two. *Ordeal* opens with, "My name is not Linda Lovelace. Not these days ... Linda Lovelace disappeared from sight several years ago."[14] The flyleaf of *Out of Bondage* similarly reads, "Linda Lovelace is nothing. The woman who used to be Linda Lovelace is here to tell you that. She doesn't exist anymore."[15]

The woman who replaces her is a deeply conservative, even Victorian, character who claims that all she ever wanted from life was, "to get married to a good man, to have children, and to someday have a home of my own."[16] She's a woman who, in order to regain her self esteem, would look in the mirror and proclaim: "Hold your head up high and remember you're a lady."[17] She's a Born-again Christian who proclaims:

"I'm a human being now so I was born again and I do believe in God."[18] She's also a prudish heterosexual, claiming she, "couldn't imagine being with another woman."[19]

Both *Ordeal* and *Out of Bondage* assert that *Inside Linda Lovelace* was really written by Chuck Traynor; indeed, they confirm that Linda Lovelace herself was his creation, thus positioning themselves as erasing the identity he created. Lovelace also discredits *The Intimate Linda Lovelace,* claiming that, "the whole book was make-believe, no better than the first one."[20] On the other hand, these two exposés, unlike the earlier book, are actually copyrighted to Linda Lovelace, alongside a man named Mike McGrady, a New York journalist who agreed to help her tell her tale. McGrady had earlier achieved fame by masterminding the group-written soft-porn sensation, *Naked Came the Stranger* (1969) and had contracted the same publisher, Lyle Stuart, to publish Lovelace's memoirs.

2.   Making Mike

The story of *Naked Came the Stranger* casts a revealing light on Lovelace's ambiguous authorship. As McGrady narrates in *Stranger Than Naked, Or How to Write Dirty Books for Fun and Profit* (1970), he and a group of male colleagues at *Newsday* conceived of the soft-core novel as a "Big Money" book in the tradition of Jacqueline Susann's *Valley of the Dolls*.[21] The book would follow the sexual exploits of a modern woman, "married, not too young, frustrated, wronged, and finally happy."[22] Each chapter would focus on one of her lovers and would be written by a different man.

After drafts of the chapters had been written, McGrady, not surprisingly, found that his heroine, a radio personality named Gillian Blake who narrates a marriage advice show with her husband, appeared differently in each chapter. His solution was ingenious. In the opening chapter he inserted a paragraph describing her in the following way:

> The major quality was something reactive, a chameleon quality that somehow enabled her to transform herself in the eyes of any man … She could become any man's dream woman, and somehow accomplish it without relinquishing her own identity.[23]

Gillian Blake, who embarks on a series of extramarital affairs upon discovering her husband's infidelity, is a somewhat paradoxical protagonist. Insofar as she is 'reactive', she becomes simply the projection of male fantasies, but through a syntactical turn ("she could become…")

granting her agency in the process, she manages to maintain a fixed identity apart from these fantasies.

Like the early Linda Lovelace, Gillian Blake represents the male fantasy of the 'liberated woman' at a crucial historical juncture when the sexual revolution is about to collide with second-wave feminism. As such, it figures the institution of marriage as constraint and the practice of adultery as liberation. Gillian and her husband William have, "an ideal marriage placed on display every morning for eight years."[24] However, the public show of their marriage masks private discontent and Gillian's affairs are meant, very much like *Deep Throat*, to represent her search for sexual fulfilment outside the conventional constraints of heterosexual monogamy. She is the fantasy of the woman who can never be satisfied by one man. The men around whom each chapter is organized - including a rabbi, an ex-boxer, a beatnik, a mobster, an abortionist, and a homosexual - present a veritable kaleidoscope of abject masculinity; men trapped in regimes of marriage, work and suburban respectability that leaves them fundamentally unable to satisfy Gillian's lust.

The most revealing chapters however, focus on authors. Chapter 11 profiles Ansel Varth, "a professional pornographer" who writes dirty books and sells them by mail order. Varth explains that he is unable to perform for Gillian since, "All I do is write books and make phone calls. I can't get it up any other way."[25] But Gillian manages to arouse him by suggesting that they "act out a story" in which she is a "lady chimpanzee" and he's "a big horny camel."[26] Their successful coupling leads him to conclude that, "he was a real man. This time he would surely write the great American dirty novel."[27] It takes the woman's agency to enable the man to translate his fantasy of masculinity into reality. Without Gillian's inspiration, Ansel Varth would remain impotent. The sexual potency she enables, translates as literary inspiration. The implication is clear - "The great American dirty novel" will be an American male fantasy of the sexually liberated American woman.

However, if Gillian enables smut, she destroys great literature. Her final lover, a hermetic author named Zoltan Caradoc who, "had already strung together enough words to more than equal the lifetime output of Proust," suffers the opposite fate of his lowbrow counterpart.[28] Caradoc is described as,

> always surrounded by the tape recorders and stereo sets
> and colour television consoles and electric typewriters.
> He lived three fourths of his life in an ultra-modern
> electronic womb. Cable umbilicals carried him regular
> progress reports from the outside world; sensitive

microphones were always handy to transmit and preserve his thoughts and memories for posterity.[29]

In the entranceway to this "electronic womb" he has a wire sculpture of himself with an erection. When Gillian arrives in his house, he warns her that "everything you say from now on will be recorded."[30] A high-tech cross between Ernest Hemingway and J.D. Salinger, Caradoc takes the literary ambition of turning life into art to its postmodern limits: "even his harshest critics agreed that he wrote from life, that this was the literature of experience."[31] If Varth, author of dirty books, spins fantasies that divorce him from the reality of his life, Caradoc, the author of classic novels, weaves the reality of his life into fantasies.

But Gillian refuses to cooperate. He tries, violently, to seduce her, but she resists his overtures, thereby destroying his literary career. After leaving his house, she receives a letter that will, "become a treasure beyond price for literary historians."[32] In it Caradoc laments that, "graduate students and scholars were going to pore over my works in the twenty-first century and write endless theses, complete with footnotes, on the identity of Zoltan Caradoc's golden goddess."[33] In refusing to cooperate she's turned the tables, and "in the end it was I who was your greatest triumph - your masterpiece of creative destruction."[34] "I had no mate, Gilly" he says in conclusion, "so you separated me from myself."[35] Caradoc's chapter ends *Naked Came the Stranger*, indicating that the male narcissism that undergirds great American literature has been irreversibly shattered by the sexually liberated American woman.

It is not at all surprising that McGrady insisted on a female author for his literary hoax. As he affirms, "it did not matter that the bulk of the book had been written by men. Penelope Ashe would be female, the more female the better."[36] Correlatively, the real male authors would represent the characters they created: in the promotional campaign for the book, each chapter was advertised with a photo of the author identified as the character. McGrady took this tack in order to ballast the authenticity of the book since, as he attests, "it is widely understood that one fairly good reason why a person would write a BM book is to make money; yet this is never admitted publicly. The stated reason is nobler - because this is a story that could not *not* be told; because the truth must out."[37] The final fantasy behind *Naked Came the Stranger* then, is that it is not a male fantasy at all, but a female reality. The 'authenticity' of Gillian Blake as a sexually liberated woman - and her lovers as pathetic men - required the legitimacy of female authorship.

The entire *Naked* hoax would seem to cast a dubious light on McGrady's collaboration with Linda Lovelace, but he had one crucial experience between the two projects which complicates their relationship considerably. In the early 70s, during the heyday of second-wave feminism, McGrady decided to quit his job at *Newsday* in order to enable his wife to pursue her independent business career. On the opening page of his memoir about the experience, titled *The Kitchen Sink Papers: My Life as a Househusband* (1975), McGrady writes, "One day, late in 1973, with all my affairs in order, I quit my job and became a housewife."[38] In the narrative that follows, McGrady shows himself becoming, "invisible, the non-essential person."[39] He laments that, "somewhere in the process I had lost track of myself and my life and my plans for a more meaningful existence."[40] He intones, "A house is not a home; it's a prison."[41] *The Kitchen Sink Papers* then becomes a sort of masculine addendum to *The Feminine Mystique*, in which McGrady confirms the empty meaninglessness of a homemaker's life. In the end his family decides to undermine conventional divisions of labour by signing on to a "private marriage contract" that distributes housework responsibilities fairly amongst all family members.[42] Flashing his new feminist credentials, McGrady concludes that, "Roles *are* reversible."[43]

However, McGrady's feminist conclusions receive one crucial qualification. At a certain point in the narrative, his wife suggests that they go see a pornographic film. Initially reluctant, McGrady agrees, but the experience is a failure. In a theatre full of men, his wife starts to giggle uncontrollably, and they have to leave right when he's getting interested. He then realizes, "not all roles can be reversed, not all experiences are interchangeable."[44] Pornography emerges as the limit case for liberal feminism's critique of the feminine mystique. It seems to prove that, when it comes to sexuality, men and women are, somehow, different. The stage is now set for McGrady's collaboration with Linda Lovelace.

3.   Creating Kitty

That stage had been set by feminism itself which, in the late 70s, increasingly took on pornography as not only a symptom but also a cause of violence against women. Women Against Violence in Pornography (WAVAM) formed in San Francisco in 1976 and Woman Against Pornography (WAP) formed in New York in 1979. In 1980, Laura Lederer released *Take Back the Night*, an influential anthology of anti-pornography feminist writings that summarized and codified this developing focus within American feminism. The philosophical underpinnings of this focus were succinctly stated by Robin Morgan: "Pornography is the theory, and rape the practice."[45] Two women - Catherine "Kitty" McKinnon and Andrea Dworkin - emerged from this consolidation of radical feminism to become the principal mouthpieces for the attack on pornography.

MacKinnon and Dworkin's writings confirm McGrady's contention that pornography functions as a limit structure in the liberal equivalence between the sexes. In her collection of essays (mostly transcripts of conference papers delivered over the preceding decade), *Feminism Unmodified* (1987), MacKinnon explains the philosophical turn whereby pornography becomes *the* crucial issue for feminists:

> Obscenity law is concerned with morality, specifically morals from the male point of view, meaning the standpoint of male dominance. The feminist critique of pornography is a politics, specifically politics from women's point of view, meaning the standpoint of the subordination of women to men. Morality here means good and evil; politics means power and powerlessness. Obscenity is a moral idea; pornography is a political practice. Obscenity is abstract; pornography is concrete.[46]

In shifting the issue from an abstract, liberal concern with free speech to a concrete, radical concern with sex discrimination, MacKinnon and Dworkin continuously return to the central substantive difference between the sexes - anatomy. Thus in her 1979 diatribe, *Pornography: Men Possessing Women,* Dworkin intones that the penis is, "the hidden symbol of terror."[47] She affirms that, "in the male system, sex is the penis, the penis is sexual power, its use in fucking is manhood."[48] Unlike the liberal feminism that had worked to achieve a basic equivalence between the sexes, Dworkin and MacKinnon continuously assert their radical difference, and that difference is always, almost obsessively, signified by the penis.

For MacKinnon, by far the more philosophically sophisticated of the two, the penis stands at the centre of a performative theory of pornography. In her high profile manifesto, *Only Words* (1993), she argues that the issue is not what pornography says, but what it does. What it does is give men erections. MacKinnon concludes that pornography, "is addressed directly to the penis, delivered through an erection, and taken out on women in the real world."[49] Indeed for MacKinnon, in the "real world" addressed by pornography, all women become victims and all men become penises.

The tour of the talk-show circuit that promoted *Ordeal* introduced Linda Lovelace to Catherine MacKinnon, who rallied to her cause, particularly after she passed a battery of lie-detector tests to prove that the brutality detailed in her book was true. Gradually, Linda Lovelace, porn queen and sexual libertarian, became Linda Marchiano, housewife and victim. Her story now became a central reference point for the anti-pornography feminists. In the 80s, she appeared at conferences with both MacKinnon and Dworkin who used her testimony in their efforts to pass anti-pornography ordinances in Minneapolis, Indianapolis, and Los Angeles. The consequences of their collaboration confirmed the degree to which pornography was coming to function as a litmus test for gender identity. As Lovelace confirmed in her last memoir, which recounts and defends her collaboration with feminists in the wake of the publicity around *Ordeal*, "women tended to believe me and most men thought I was lying."[50]

Nevertheless, the relatively easy oppositions of Lovelace's conversion - from pleasure to pain, from free agent to trapped victim, from male fantasy to feminist reality - are complicated by the very event on which they turn - the enormous popularity of *Deep Throat* and the subsequent superstardom of Linda Lovelace. The success of *Deep Throat* catapulted Lovelace into the media limelight, surrounding her with social opportunities that threatened Traynor's authority over her. As she concedes in the later confessional texts, the confidence and connections she gained from her fame finally enabled her to escape from his clutches.

In this sense, the most revealing, and dialectically complex, of her autobiographies is *The Intimate Diary*, which opens with an extended meditation on celebrity. Thus she affirms, "The most marketable thing in this country is a well-known name. My name can sell shoes or help publicize someone's porno crackdown."[51] She astutely notes that the two primary cultural functions of this name are indicated by the subpoena and the autograph. Indeed, a key moment in the text occurs when the man serving her a subpoena asks for her autograph for his niece: "I signed my name with a little heart over the 'i' like I always do and watched him walk away" she says, "I had the subpoena and he had his autograph. I didn't come out too well on that exchange, I thought, but at least he went away happy."[52]

This trivial yet symptomatic exchange of the subpoena for the autograph indicates how Lovelace's celebrity enables her complex evidentiary role in the politicised battles over pornography. The currency of her fame heightened the value of her testimony during the anti-pornography backlash of the late 70s and early 80s. MacKinnon comments on the crucial role of such testimony by exposing the underlying politics of pornography:

> Once abused women are heard and ... become real,
> women's silence can no longer be the context in which
> pornography and speech are analyzed ... Instead of the

forces of darkness seeking to suppress what the forces of
light are struggling to free, her captivity itself is put in
issue for the first time ... Before, each woman who said
she was abused looked incredible and exceptional; now,
the abuse appears deadeningly commonplace. Before,
what was done to her was sex; now, it is sexual abuse.
Before, she was sex; now, she is a human being
gendered female - if anyone can figure out what that is.[53]

Not only does such testimony shift the grounds of the debate from a moral
issue over the nature of obscenity to a political issue over the nature of
sexual subordination, it, in essence, generates gender difference as such: it
creates the "human being gendered female," who, for MacKinnon, is
centrally signified by the victim of sexual abuse.

Correlatively, pornography should reveal the nature of the abuser,
the human being gendered male. A viewing of *Deep Throat* reveals the
ambiguous accuracy of MacKinnon and Dworkin's claims in this regard.
As a narrative thematically oriented around fellatio, it is, like most porn
oriented toward male viewers, obsessed with the erect penis. However, the
penis is, if anything, more disembodied and objectified than Lovelace's
own ambiguous sexuality. In the opening credits, the male roles are
introduced by numbers, while Linda Lovelace is introduced "as Herself."
The film begins with Lovelace's rotation through multiple partners in her
search for sexual pleasure, and concludes with her becoming a
"physiotherapist" helping men with sexual dysfunctions. As in most
pornography, the men are rigorously reduced to their sex organs and their
ability to achieve and maintain an erection. In essence, the men are penises
and numbers, the woman is a face and a name. Indeed, summarizing
Behind the Green Door, another exemplar of porn's Golden Age,
Williams comments on the, "abundance of interchangeable men - and their
penises - in relation to a single woman." As Williams affirms, this tends to
be the plot structure of feature-length porn from this era.[54]

It is in this double reduction, I believe, that we can see how the
contemporary culture of celebrity provides a link between pornography
and feminism in the wake of their overlapping heydays, and indeed shows
how MacKinnon herself has been able to leverage status as a celebrity
feminist through her attack on pornography. On one hand, men are posited
as anonymous masturbators; on the other, women are posited as private
victims whose stories must be made public. MacKinnon locates herself as
the mouth through whom her victims speak and pornography becomes the
male penis that is trying to shut her up, for as she claims, "who listens to a
woman with a penis in her mouth?"[55]

As Jennifer Wicke has noted, with the decline of movement feminism in the late70s, celebrity became, "a new locus for feminist discourse, feminist politics, and feminist conflicts."[56] Wicke affirms that "MacKinnon is set squarely in the celebrity zone and looks likely to stay there for the time being."[57] It is more than coincidental that this new celebrity feminism has taken on pornography as one of its key issues. For celebrity, like pornography, works on the assumption that the individual body on public display can metonymically channel the desires and needs of an anonymous audience. They both assume that we can only overcome our private impotence through witnessing the performance of public figures.

As the volatile reception of *Only Words* revealed, it is MacKinnon's celebrity that underpins her fixation on gender difference. In his provocative review for the *Nation*, "Between the Motion and the Act," Carlin Romano imagined raping MacKinnon as an exercise in testing the thesis of her book: are pornographic words the same as sexual acts? MacKinnon took the bait, arguing that Romano's review amounted to "a public rape" by which "all women are hurt."[58] As Romano undoubtedly intended, her angry response exposed the philosophical absurdity of her ideas, but it also confirmed a reality about celebrity culture: for a star (and Romano affirms that "MacKinnon is on a star trip"[59]) public image is as real as private experience. If Romano "hurt" MacKinnon's public self he did, in a sense, hurt her.

In hurting her, he also affirmed her need to represent "all women" as victims of male violence. Romano asserts that her Cartesian creed can be translated as "I am raped, therefore I am."[60] As many of her critics agree, MacKinnon needs the very sexism she decries in order to leverage her role as public spokeswoman for all women. Thus Wendy Brown, in her excellent essay "The Mirror of Pornography," states that,

> MacKinnon's theory of gender transpires within a pornographic genre, suspending us in a complex of pornographic experience in which MacKinnon is both purveyor and object of desire and her analysis is proffered as substitute for the sex she abuses us for wanting.[61]

Brown effectively reveals the degree to which MacKinnon's writing mirrors the pornographic imagination she vilifies. What Brown neglects to emphasize, in my opinion, is the degree to which MacKinnon's celebrity is, in essence, the "mirror" which enables the symmetry between feminism and pornography. She can only be "purveyor and object of desire" in a public sphere that enables her to circulate as the figure not only for all women, but also for the very sign of sex as the ultimate reality of gender.

In this public sphere, MacKinnon's engagement with Linda Lovelace figures as a reaction formation to the failure of both pornography and feminism to effectively represent, and liberate, women as a unified category of person. Both pornography and feminism in the early 70s effectively challenged traditional American protocols of representing female power and pleasure by breaking down the boundaries between public and private, and both initially envisioned a utopian sense of liberation as the consequence of the challenges they posed. Pornography did enable franker public discussion of sex, and feminism did transform the protocols of gender relations, but the different liberations each envisioned failed to ensue. Rather, new contradictions emerged between sexual pleasure and sexual power in the public sphere. Celebrity performances like the relationship between Catherine MacKinnon and Linda Lovelace, as a contained enactment of the interpenetration of public and private, function as symptoms of these new contradictions.

Notes

1. On *Miller v. California* and the censorship battles that led up to it, see de Grazia, 561-72. For the effect of *Miller v. California* on the hard-core film industry, see Lewis, 192-230.
2. For an excellent overview of this ongoing debate, see Cornell.
3. On the utility of the term "public subject" for an understanding of contemporary celebrity, see Marshall, 251.
4. See, in particular, Marshall, 203-50.
5. For a Foucaultian take on the epistemological nature of porn as a component of the modern "knowledge-pleasure" regime, see Williams, 2-9.
6. Lovelace, 1973, flyleaf.
7. Ibid., 51.
8. Ibid., 19.
9. Ibid,. 21.
10. Ibid., 32.
11. Ibid., 52.
12. Lovelace, 1974, 8.
13. Ibid., frontispiece.
14. Lovelace, 1980, 1.
15. Lovelace, 1986, flyleaf.
16. Lovelace, 1980, 72.
17. Lovelace, 1986, 36.

18. Ibid., 178.
19. Lovelace, 1980, 51.
20. Ibid., 249.
21. McGrady, 1970, 2.
22. Ibid., 16.
23. Ashe, 1969, 13.
24. Ibid., 12.
25. Ibid., 173.
26. Ibid.
27. Ibid., 174.
28. Ibid., 208.
29. Ibid.
30. Ibid., 211.
31. Ibid., 210.
32. Ibid., 214-5.
33. Ibid., 217.
34. Ibid., 215.
35. Ibid., 217.
36. McGrady, 1970, 62.
37. Ibid., 134.
38. McGrady, 1975, 1.
39. Ibid., 57.
40. Ibid,. 60.
41. Ibid., 57.
42. Ibid., 181.
43. Ibid., 166.
44. Ibid., 132.
45. Lederer, 1980, 139.
46. MacKinnon, 1987, 147.
47. Dworkin, 1979, 15.
48. Ibid., 23.
49. MacKinnon, 2000, 104.
50. Lovelace and McGrady, 1986, 113.
51. Lovelace, 1974, 4.
52. Ibid., 5.
53. MacKinnon, 2000, 97.
54. Williams, 1989, 159.
55. MacKinnon, 1987, 193.
56. Wicke, 1994, 753.
57. Ibid., 774.
58. Cited in Streitfeld, 1994, 7.
59. Romano, 1993, 564.

60. Ibid., 564.
61. Brown, 2000, 211

References

Ashe. P. (1969), *Naked Came the Stranger.* New York: Dell.

Brown, B. (2000), 'The Mirror of Pornography', in: Cornell (ed.), 198-217

Cornell, D. (ed.) (2000), *Feminism and Pornography.* New York: Oxford UP.

Damian, G. (director). (1972), *Deep Throat.* [film]. Arrow Films. USA.

Dworkin, A. (1979), *Pornography: Men Possessing Women.* New York: Plume.

Herlihy, J. L. (1968), *Midnight cowboy.* London: Panther.

Lewis, J. (2000), *Hollywood v. Hard Core: How the Struggle over Censorship Saved the Modern Film Industry.* New York: NYU Press.

Lovelace, L. (1974), *The Intimate Diary of Linda Lovelace.* New York: Pinnacle.

Lovelace, L. (1973), *Inside Linda Lovelace.* New York: Pinnacle.

Lovelace, L. (With M. McGrady) (1986), *Out of Bondage.* Secaucus: Lyle Stuart.

Lovelace, L. (With M. McGrady) (1980), *Ordeal.* New York: Berkeley.
MacKinnon, C. (1987), *Feminism Unmodified: Discourses on Life and Law.* Cambridge: Harvard UP.

MacKinnon, C. (2000), 'Only Words', in: D. Cornell, (ed.) (2000), *Feminism and Pornography.* New York: Oxford UP.

Marshall, P. (1997), *Celebrity and Power: Fame in Contemporary Culture.* Minneapolis: U of Minnesota P.

McGrady, M. (1970), *Stranger Than Naked, Or How to Write Dirty Books for Fun and Profit.* New York: Peter H. Wyden.

McGrady, M. (1975), *The Kitchen Sink Papers: My Life as a Househusband.* New York: Doubleday.

Romano, C. (1993), 'Between the Motion and the Act', *The Nation*, 257: 563-70.

Roth, P. (1969), *Portnoy's Complaint.* New York: Random House.

Wicke, J. (1994), 'Celebrity Material: Materialist Feminism and the Culture of Celebrity', *South Atlantic Quarterly* 93: 751-78.

Williams, L. (1989), *Hard Core: Power, Pleasure, and the "Frenzy of the Visible."* Berkeley: U of California P.

"Video Abuse":
Gender, Censorship and *I Spit on Your Grave*

Darren Oldridge

In a stirring editorial in the summer of 1983, *The Daily Mail* urged the newly re-elected government of Margaret Thatcher to confront an insidious social evil. Recalling the "gin-soaked brutality" of 18th century London, it asked if "the video shops of today" were any less "squalid or corrupting than the gin alleys of two centuries ago". Drawing out the metaphor, *The Mail* noted that "there had to be laws to limit alcohol abuse, and there must be a law now ... to fight video abuse."[1] The belief that violent videos were like drugs was not confined to the British tabloids. The introduction to the government report on 'video nasties' in 1985 claimed that their makers and distributors were no better than drug-dealers and should be placed under similar legal restraints.[2] If violent movies were like drugs, then the most toxic of them all was *I Spit on Your Grave*. The film featured heavily in the press campaign against 'video nasties' between 1982 and 1984, and its most infamous scene probably inspired the title of *The Mail*'s editorial: 'Rape of Our Children's Minds'. Directed by Meir Zarchi in 1978, *I Spit on Your Grave* tells the story of a woman subjected to gang rape who takes revenge on her attackers. Although it has rarely been screened, Zarchi's movie continues to provoke extreme reactions from both critics and censors. This chapter will offer a new evaluation of the picture and its extraordinary reception in the last twenty years.

Released at the start of the boom in home video, *I Spit on Your Grave* was one of the first films to secure commercial success through the new medium. The picture fared badly at the American box office, but took off on the video market, reaching number 24 in *Billboard*'s list of best selling titles for 1981.[3] Zarchi's picture was never shown in cinemas in the UK, but was available on video until 1984, when its distributors were forced to withdraw it under the terms of the Video Recordings Act. The movie was denied a certificate until February 2002, when the British Board of Film Classification permitted a heavily cut version to be re-issued on video.

From the time of its US release, the critical response to *I Spit* has been crushingly negative. Indeed Peter Lehman, one of the film's few defenders, has called Zarchi's movie "one of the most reviled films of all time".[4] It is hard to dispute this verdict. The veteran American critic, Roger Ebert, offered a visceral account of his response to the film:

> *I Spit on Your Grave* is a vile bag of garbage that is so

sick, reprehensible and contemptible that I can hardly
believe that it played in respectable theatres. But it did.
Attending it was one of the most depressing experiences
of my life ... At the film's end I walked out of the
theatre   quickly,   feeling   unclean,   ashamed   and
depressed.[5]

To Mick Martin and Marsha Porter, *I Spit* is "an utterly reprehensible
motion picture with shockingly misplaced values . . . one of the most
tasteless, irresponsible and disturbing movies ever made".[6] More
succinctly, Kim Newman dismissed the picture as one of "the most
loathsome films of all time".[7] On its UK video release this year, Mark
Dinning, the reviewer in *Empire* magazine, called it a "vile, odious little
haemorrhoid".[8]

The censors have echoed these extreme reactions. In Britain, *I
Spit* was one of the first videos to be prosecuted under the Obscene
Publications Act, along with *Driller Killer* and *Death Trap*. As a result,
the police removed 234 copies of Zarchi's film from the offices of Astra
Video in May 1982.[9] Even in the more liberal atmosphere of the early 21st
century, it was one of the last 'nasties' to be granted a certificate by the
British Board of Film Classification, years after titles like *The Evil Dead*,
The Driller Killer and *Cannibal Holocaust*. Moreover, the Board insisted
on seven minutes of cuts before allowing the re-issue of Zarchi's movie.
The Driller Killer in contrast, was cut by just fifty-four seconds. Unlike
other films proscribed by the Video Recordings Act, *I Spit on Your Grave*
has received only half-hearted support from opponents of censorship.
Some such critics have viewed the film as an embarrassment. Trevor
Mathews for example, identifies *I Spit* as one of the "tawdry examples of
the cinema" that caused other, superior films to be tarred "with the 'nasty'
brush".[10] Remarkably, Mark Dinning's review in *Empire* applauds the
BBFC for its severe censorship: "We should just be grateful", he
concludes, that "this release has actually been trimmed."[11]

This extraordinary response cries out for serious attention. If
critical opinion or censorship provides any measure of contemporary
attitudes towards the media, the peculiar infamy of Zarchi's movie merits
careful examination. The need for such scrutiny is even more urgent for
the small minority of viewers who regard *I Spit on Your Grave* as a good
film. One of the striking aspects of the picture's history is that very few
critics have attempted to defend it on artistic grounds. A notable exception
is Marco Starr, who claimed in 1984 that the film was "well made,
interestingly   written,   beautifully   photographed   and   intelligently
directed".[12] The first part of this chapter will attempt to confirm Starr's

judgement. Despite its appalling reputation, *I Spit* is a clever and effective piece of filmmaking, which challenges many of the conventions of the horror *genre*. This assessment prompts some obvious questions about the film's reception. These will be addressed in the second part, which argues that the film's unusually thoughtful treatment of gender and sexual violence provoked a backlash from male critics and guardians of public morality.

1.   The Film

For viewers aware of its fearful reputation, watching the uncut *I Spit on Your Grave* is an odd experience. The movie's press has been so aggressively hostile - and contains so many inaccuracies - that the picture itself feels like a different film. The British media campaign against *I Spit* established several myths about its contents, and these were perpetuated in the government working party report on video violence in 1985. The appendix to this report contains a garbled account of the film's plot, featuring several distortions and one completely non-existent scene. Candidly, the authors acknowledge that this information was obtained without viewing the film. Instead, it was put together from "trade descriptions in video magazines and journals, descriptions on the boxes of video cassettes, and synopses that have been presented in court as evidence by the prosecution."[13] Several misleading reports about the picture continue to circulate. To cut through this thicket of misinformation, it is necessary to provide a brief outline of the film.

The movie opens with Jennifer Hills (Camille Keaton), an aspiring writer leaving New York for a summer's retreat in the country. Here she attempts to compose her first novel, but finds her work disturbed by a gang of local men. Three of them capture her in the woods outside her rented cabin, and egg on a fourth man named Matthew to rape her. Matthew is plainly scared and intimidated by the situation. He refuses to penetrate Jennifer but assists the others in her rape. The gang release Jennifer and she wanders into the forest. Here she encounters the men again, and is raped once more. They abandon Jennifer on a rock and she stumbles back to her cabin. The men are lying in wait and she is raped for a third time. As the gang departs, Matthew is bullied by the others to kill Jennifer with a knife. He lets her live but tells his friends that he has murdered her. The picture now shifts gear. Jennifer recovers painfully from her ordeal and renews work on the book. She visits a church and asks God to forgive her for the actions she is planning. She returns to the rented house and orders groceries from a local store where Matthew works as a deliveryman. When he arrives, Jennifer tempts him into the forest, seduces him, slips a rope around his neck and hangs him from a tree. Next she picks up Johnny, the gang leader, and forces him to strip at gunpoint. In a remarkable sequence, Johnny apparently persuades her to drop the gun: she admits that she finds him attractive and invites him back to the cabin. They take a bath together and she stabs his genitals. After locking him in the bathroom, she listens to classical music as he bleeds to death. The last two rapists ride out to the cabin in a powerboat. Jennifer ambushes the boat, kills one of the men with an axe, and cuts up the other with the boat's propeller. She rides away with a hard smile on her face.

The most controversial scenes in the movie are the three rapes. These scenes have been frequently misrepresented. To take one example, Kim Newman stated in 1988 that "the rape lasts an unbearable, demeaning 45 minutes."[14] Mark Dinning repeated this claim in *Empire* in 2002.[15] This is simply false: there are three separate rapes, and the sequence from the first attack to the last is less than 25 minutes. Other commentators have suggested that Jennifer appears to enjoy the rapes.[16] This is also untrue. In fact, it is hard to imagine a more extreme misrepresentation of the film. One of the most striking qualities of Zarchi's picture is its total identification with Jennifer during the rape sequences. From *Friday the 13th* (1980) onwards, 'slasher' films in the 1980s conventionally employed a 'subjective camera' to present the viewpoint of the killer. Some critics have condemned this trend for encouraging audiences to identify with the murderer against his victims. Almost uniquely, *I Spit on Your Grave* uses the subjective camera to show Jennifer's viewpoint as she flees her attackers. When she is finally held down, the camera cuts repeatedly from her screaming face to the brutal expressions of the men bearing down on her. The effect is extremely distressing, as the viewer is forced to identify with a victim of appalling sexual violence. As Carol Clover has noted, "not for a moment does she express anything but protest, fear and pain."[17] Zarchi's sympathy for Jennifer is underlined by a medium-range shot of her discarded body after the second rape; the camera holds this shot as the rapists amble off into the woods, and fixes it for several seconds after they have gone. Few people watching this scene could dispute Marco Starr's observation that "the rapists in *I Spit on Your Grave* believe that abused women should be thrown away and forgotten; the film-maker quite definitely does not."[18]

It is easy enough to counter the allegation that *I Spit* condones sexual violence. Several academic writers have made this point, though the myth that Zarchi's movie is an 'exploitation' film persists in the mainstream media. Few critics however, have gone beyond this to argue that *I Spit* is an artistic success. Carol Clover describes it as derivative and "roughly made."[19] In a recent review of the films at the centre of the UK 'video nasties' controversy, Andrew Holmes points out that Zarchi's picture does not deserve to be listed alongside such crude and bloodthirsty titles as *Maniac* (1980) and *The Beast in Heat* (1977): nonetheless, his article describes the film as an exploitation picture overlaid with an insincere "message".[20] The view that *I Spit* is a serious and effective work of art is, of course, a subjective judgement. There is no way for me to prove this claim and I accept that many readers will dismiss it, but I can at least suggest that there are good reasons for seeing the film in this way. An examination of two key scenes should make the point. Both come from the second half of the film, which has generally attracted less attention than the notorious rape sequences. Indeed, it is one of the many injustices to Zarchi's movie that the controversy over the rapes has diverted attention from the complex and beautifully composed episodes that follow.

The first scene to consider is Matthew's murder. The sequence begins in the grocery store, where Matthew is told to make the delivery to Jennifer's cabin. As he contemplates this news, he stares across the counter to where a plucked chicken is being splayed and cut into pieces. He conceals a knife in his pocket and sets off with the order. As he approaches the house, Jennifer steps from the woods in a white dress. She beckons him and he follows her nervously into the forest, holding out the knife. She leads him to a tree beside the river, where he approaches her with the knife raised in a trembling hand. Unafraid, she calls him closer and begins to unbutton her dress. He drops the knife, apparently frozen with fear and desire. She pulls him to the ground and they start to make love. As he moves above her, Jennifer produces a noose from behind the tree and drops it over his head. She tugs the other end of the rope and pulls him upright, then levers the rope against a branch to heave his whole body off the ground. His body swings out over the river and the camera closes in on his twitching face.

This is, without doubt, a deeply unpleasant sequence. But the events are also realised with a strange poetry. Jennifer appears invulnerable and ghost-like; indeed, the whole scene in the woods has the feel of a supernatural tale. This atmosphere is shaped by the sense of impending horror that surrounds Matthew as he prepares to visit the cabin, by Jennifer's sudden appearance dressed in white, and the otherworldly logic of the events themselves. The idea of Jennifer as an avenging spirit is established by the preceding narrative, in which she is apparently killed and returns to life. The fact that Matthew is the first victim of her revenge gives the scene a further poignancy: it was his act that effectively brought her back from the dead. Matthew's murder also underlines the remorseless nature of Jennifer's revenge. As the reluctant accomplice in the rapes, he was the least culpable member of the gang. If his killing had occurred later in the film, it may well have suggested that Jennifer's sense of justice was ebbing. By killing Matthew first, Zarchi confronts the audience with the terrible impartiality of his heroine's actions. Since we have already viewed the appalling rapes from Jennifer's perspective, we understand her decision to kill Matthew, but we also perceive that her act may be unjust. This makes the murder particularly troubling. The viewer's sense of unease is magnified by a third element in the sequence; the combination of seduction, sex and execution. Writing from a psychoanalytical perspective, Barbara Creed has argued that Matthew's murder portrays a misogynistic connection between women, sex and death.[21] But a simpler and more positive reading is possible. The erotic nature of the killing can be seen as an affirmation of Jennifer's power. She uses her sexual attractiveness literally to disarm Matthew. Moreover, his execution during their lovemaking is a crudely poetic revenge for his participation in the rapes. Taken together, these elements create one of the most disturbing sequences in modern horror cinema; and its intricate construction suggests that the unnerving power of the sequence is no accident.

The intensity of the events leading to Matthew's death are matched by the scene where Jennifer confronts Johnny, the gang leader, and makes him strip at gunpoint. This, again, is a striking demonstration of her determination and control, but in this case a confident and charismatic victim challenges her power. Kneeling and naked, Johnny offers a blustering defence of the rapes:

> C'mon. This thing with you is a thing that any man
> would have done. You coax a man into doing it, a man
> gets the message fast. Whether a man is married or not,
> he's still a man. Hey, first thing, you come into the gas
> station and you expose your damn sexy legs to me,
> walking back and forth real slow, making sure I see
> them good. And then Matthew delivers the food to your
> door. He sees half your tits peeking out at him, tits with
> no bra. And then you're lying in your canoe, in your
> bikini, like bait.

Johnny's words are undercut by the humiliating context in which he is forced to express them, but his courage and obvious confidence in his physical attractiveness also lend him a certain authority. This is apparently confirmed in the climactic sequence, when he holds out his hand and Jennifer surrenders the gun. Here the sexual power game is extremely taut: Johnny appears to have won, and could easily use the gun to assert his mastery, but instead he submits to Jennifer's promise of sex. At this point her victory is total, and the audience is painfully aware that his fate is sealed.

Both these sequences demonstrate one of the most striking characteristics of *I Spit on Your Grave*. This is its tendency to invert cinematic conventions, both in terms of plot and composition. When Jennifer drops the gun into Johnny's hand, she re-enacts a scene familiar from many other crime films: an emotional attacker is disarmed by the words of a brave and perceptive hero. But Johnny, of course, is not the hero of this piece, and Jennifer's apparent surrender only confirms her power. Likewise, the scene where Matthew brandishes a knife as he follows Jennifer into the woods echoes countless 'slasher' films of the late 1970s and early 1980s, but Matthew is destined to be the victim, not the killer. Zarchi's use of music also subverts the conventions of film. The first 20 minutes of *I Spit* have no music at all. This makes the picture feel like a documentary, and adds to the trauma of the first rape. Then a harmonica solo drifts through the forest as Jennifer walks naked from the scene of her ordeal. For a moment, it seems that the picture has become 'safe'; the music distances the audience from the realistic depiction of the assault and its aftermath. As Jennifer steps into a clearing however, we see that Andy, one of the rapists, is playing the harmonica. The music is part of the 'live action' of the film. He continues to play as his friends emerge from behind the trees, and his melody quickens as they pursue their victim. Such subversive effects confirm the view of David Kerekes and David Slater that Zarchi's film is "very anti-cinema".[22] They also indicate the director's intelligence and willingness to upset the expectations of his audience.

Among the many deliberately unsettling elements in Zarchi's film is his portrayal of its heroine. Camille Keaton's character is unique in cinema: she is a sane and intelligent female rape survivor who gets away with murder. In the last part of this chapter, I will argue that this is one of the reasons for the extremely hostile response to the film from the critics and censors.

2.   The Film's Reception

It is curious that *I Spit on Your Grave*, a film often described as 'pornographic', appears to be disliked most intensely by members of the social group that normally consume pornography - men. From Roger Ebert's call to filmgoers to boycott cinemas that showed the picture on its release to Mark Dinning's contemptuous review in 2002, male critics have voiced the most violent condemnations of the movie. During the British 'video nasties' controversy in 1983-4, it was also male campaigners and politicians who took the lead in denouncing the film. In part, of course, this reflects the dominance of men in the media and politics: most reviewers of *all* films are men, and the British government and opposition parties were even more male-dominated in the early 1980s than they are today. There are, nonetheless, good reasons to assume that men find Zarchi's movie particularly distressing. As Camille Keaton herself noted in 1982, the film makes "males in the audience singularly uncomfortable".[23]

Why should this be? The observation that *I Spit* particularly troubles men suggests that the murders may be one source of anxiety. Exceptionally for a horror film, a woman commits all the killings, and her victims are all male. Peter Lehman has drawn attention to this aspect of the film, suggesting that the sexualised murders touch on male fears of repressed homosexuality.[24] Barbara Creed also focuses on the murder scenes, and claims that they dramatise the male fear of castration by a woman.[25] Both of these readings depend heavily on psychoanalysis and stand or fall on the reliability of this approach. A simpler explanation perhaps, is that male viewers rarely see films that depict men in states of abject terror.[26] From the earliest days of film, the image of the terrified woman has been a cinematic staple. Male terror in the face of death is far less common. Such terror in the context of sexual murder is rarer still. This aspect of *I Spit* may, then, account for some extreme responses to the film. The sexual mutilation of men is also a cinematic rarity, and appears to evoke particular horror in some reviewers. Martin and Porter for example, describe Johnny's apparent castration in the bath as "one of the most appalling moments in cinema history".[27] Other writers have claimed falsely that Johnny's friends are castrated as well. Thus the British government report on 'video nasties' contains this odd description of the final murder: "the woman starts the engine of a boat when the blades are in his genital area, apparently castrating him and leaving his body covered in blood in the river".[28] Similarly, Mark Dinning claims that Jennifer "mutilates the gonads of the perpetrators [of her rape] beyond repair."[29] In fact, only Johnny suffers an assault to his genitals. Moreover, the act itself takes place off camera, and it is by no means clear that he has been castrated. Here it seems that male viewers of Zarchi's movie have been scared by their own imaginations.

Another feature of the murders that may be problematic for a male audience is the character of their perpetrator. In popular fiction and news reports, female killers tend to be classified within a limited range of types: they are either accomplices to men, victims of 'hysteria' or PMS, or driven to murder in the heat of passion or rage. Those who do not conform easily to these categories, such as Myra Hindley, are presented as uncommonly evil.[30] The heroine of *I Spit on Your Grave* evades all the conventional models for a woman who kills. She is clearly driven by revenge, but her revenge is premeditated to an exceptional degree. Each murder is elaborately planned and the first two involve luring the victim to the place of his death. The killings are not carried out in anger; rather, she toys coolly with the men until the moment of their despatch. Jennifer is plainly not mad: she finds ingenious ways to overpower her victims and takes meticulous care in concealing her crimes. The critic Phil Hardy has noted how "the film distances the viewer" from Keaton's character during the murder sequences.[31] This is hardly surprising, since Zarchi ignores all the normal rules for depicting a female killer. After the horror of the rapes, we *want* to be on her side, but her actions have no place within the acceptable range of female behaviour. For female viewers this scenario is potentially liberating. For men, it is more likely to create feelings of alienation.

While its depiction of the sexual murder of men has probably contributed to the vilification of *I Spit on Your Grave*, it is the rape scenes that have been the focus of most condemnation. Here the critics' arguments are revealingly confused. It has often been claimed that the film cynically exploits violence against women. Roger Ebert, for example, denounced *I Spit* in 1982 as "the worst of the summer's exploitation films", with a "sick attitude towards women."[32] This claim would be plausible if Zarchi's movie showed no sympathy for its rape victim, trivialised her suffering, or presented it as entertainment. But this is not so. Arguably, Stanley Kubrick's *A Clockwork Orange* (1971) could be condemned on these grounds, since the rapes in Kubrick's film are viewed mainly from the perpetrators' perspective, with little acknowledgement of the victims' suffering. *A Clockwork Orange*, however, enjoys a strong critical reputation and was passed uncut by the British censors.[33] The main problem with the rapes in *I Spit* is precisely the opposite of Ebert's claim: they show the effects of male sexual violence in unflinching detail and invite the audience to participate in the suffering they cause. In other words, they are *too horrible*. Paradoxically, this fact has been acknowledged by most of the film's detractors, who describe the rapes as "unbearable" or "repulsive". It also appears that the horror of the rape scenes was the main concern of the British censors. When a legal version of the video appeared in 2002, the cuts imposed by the British Board of Film Classification removed many of the shots of Camille Keaton's screaming face during the rapes. Indeed, all such images were expunged from the second rape scene: here Keaton's body is completely absent, leaving only the faces of her attackers on screen. The result is a strangely abstract and dehumanised sequence, redeemed only by Zarchi's memorable shot of Keaton's body abandoned on the rock. The scene where Jennifer walks back to the cabin, bloody and smeared with dirt, has also been cut. The effect of these interventions is to reduce the awfulness of her ordeal and divert attention from its consequences.

The sheer horror of the rapes then, helps to explain their violent condemnation by some men. Another factor may also contribute to this reaction: the circumstances in which the attacks are portrayed. The rape sequences in *I Spit* explicitly renounce many common myths about male sexual violence. These include the idea that women can enjoy rape, that 'no' sometimes means 'yes', that some women invite assault by their provocative behaviour or clothes, that men are subject to sudden, uncontainable sexual urges, and that rapes are normally committed by strangers. Zarchi's film flatly rejects all of these views. The first myth is obviously challenged by the attacks themselves. Subsequently, Jennifer exploits the rapists' belief that she "really liked it" in order to kill them. This is how she gets Johnny into her car and later persuades him to join her in the bath. Indeed, Johnny's murder can be read as a vicious joke that deliberately subverts the myth: Jennifer appears to masturbate him before slipping a knife under the water and as she continues to touch him - either with her hand or the knife - he says: "God bless your hands ... that's so sweet ... that's so sweet it's painful". The film also repudiates the idea that women can provoke sexual attacks by their dress or behaviour. Jennifer clearly wears a bikini for comfort, not to display herself to men, and when the attacks begin, she resists them with all her strength. Equally, the rapists in *I Spit* are not suddenly overwhelmed by irresistible impulses: all the attacks are premeditated and the last one is a carefully staged ambush. Finally, the assailants are not strangers: Jennifer spends time with Johnny and Matthew in the opening scenes of the film. The complete refusal of Zarchi's movie to acknowledge any of these myths about rape contrasts with other films in the rape-revenge *genre*, including some that have been praised for their sensitive and 'responsible' treatment of sexual violence. In *Lipstick* (1976), for example, there is some ambiguity about the heroine's responsibility for her rape. The same can be said of *The Accused* (1988), which also suggests that the rapists were impelled by spontaneous sexual drives.

One last reason for the extreme condemnation of the rape scenes in *I Spit* may be the subversive, 'anti-cinema' approach of Zarchi's filmmaking. Discarding the conventions for depicting sex on screen, he plays out the rapes in what seems to be real time, with static cameras, and no music. Even without violence, this approach would discomfort most audiences. Only those familiar with pornography would have any frame of reference for the events on screen and this would be wholly inappropriate for a mainstream movie. As Kerekes and Slater point out, *I Spit* employs pornographic conventions to unsettle its viewers.[34] It is hardly surprising that men in particular should feel defensive and troubled by this. Since the scenes involve brutal and coercive sex, male viewers unnerved by them are likely to respond in two ways: they can trivialise them with laughter, or condemn them as 'violent pornography'. The second option is appealing as it distances men from the suggestion that 'normal' pornography should be condemned. Occasionally, this fear is explicit in reviews of the film. Thus Alan Jones offered this comment in 1982:

> The protracted rape is … as degrading and squirm-inducing as anything I've seen in the exploitation field … This irresponsibility would give the 'violence against women' lobby enough ammunition to successfully campaign against anything they wished to.[35]

In practice, it appears that the "squirm-inducing" qualities of Zarchi's picture have provoked male critics and censors to denounce it as the worst kind of pornography. With a sad irony, it appears that the subversive qualities that make *I Spit on Your Grave* such a clever film have also contributed to its evil reputation.

Notes

1. Barlow and Hill, 1985, 6.
2. Barker, 1984a, 28.
3. Kerekes and Slater, 2000, 189
4. Lehman, 1993, 103.
5. Ebert, 1989, 360.
6. Martin and Porter, 1987, 704.
7. Newman, 1988, 57.
8. Dinning, 2002, 131.
9. Kerekes and Slater, 2000, 40.
10. Mathews, 1994, 249.
11. Dinning, 131.
12. Starr, 1984, 49.
13. Barlow and Hill, 175.
14. Newman, 1988, 57.
15. Dinning, 131.
16. This claim was made during a British rape trial in June 1983 and reported uncritically by some sections of the press. See Barker, 1984b, 113-4.
17. Clover, 1992, 118; see also Hardy, 1986, 329.
18. Starr, 52.

19. Clover, 118.
20. Holmes, 2002, 12.
21. Creed, 1993, 129-30.
22. Kerekes and Slater, 191.
23. Starr, 54.
24. Lehman, 1993, 103-17.
25. Creed, 128-31.
26. Carol Clover makes this point forcefully, and cites *I Spit on Your Grave* as a revealing exception. Clover, 51.
27. Martin and Porter, 704.
28. Barlow and Hill, 179.
29. Dinning, 131.
30. Hardy, 1986, 329.
31. See Barker, forthcoming; also Birch, 1993, 32-61.
32. Ebert, 1981.
33. *A Clockwork Orange* was released without cuts in the UK in January 1972. It was subsequently withdrawn by its director Stanley Kubrick, but was re-released uncut after his death in 2000.
34. Kerekes and Slater, 191.
35. Starr, 49.

References

Barker, M. (1984a), 'Nasty Politics or Video Nasties?', in: M. Barker, (ed.), *The Video Nasties: Freedom and Censorship in the Media*. London: Pluto, 7-38.

Barker, M. (1984b), 'Nasties: A Problem of Identification', in: M. Barker (ed.), *The Video Nasties: Freedom and Censorship in the Media*. London: Pluto, 104-18.

Barker, M. (Forthcoming), 'Women, Children and the Myth of Evil', in: D. Medlicott and S. Morris (eds.). *Territories of Evil*. London: Rodopi

Barlow, G. and A. Hill (eds.) (1985), *Video Violence and Children*. London: Hodder and Stoughton.

Batzella, L. (director). (1977), *The Beast in Heat*. [film]. Eterna Film. Italy.

Birch, H. (1993), 'If Looks could Kill: Myra Hindley and the Iconography of Evil', in: H. Birch (ed.), *Moving Targets: Women, Murder and*

Representation. London: Virago.

Clover, C. J. (1992), *Men, Women and Chainsaws: Gender in the Modern Horror Film*. Princeton: Princeton University Press.

Creed, B. (1993), *The Monstrous Feminine: Film, Feminism, Psychoanalysis*. London: Routledge.

Cunningham, S. S. (director). (1980), *Friday the 13th*. [film] Georgetown Productions Inc., Paramount Pictures and Sean S. Cunningham Films. USA.

Deodato, R. (director). (1979), *Cannibal Holocaust*. [film]. F.D. Cinematografica. Colombia and Italy

Dinning, M. (2002), review in *Empire*, March, 131.

Ebert, R. (1981), 'Why American Audiences Aren't Safe Anymore', *American Film*, March, 55.

Ebert, R. (1989), *Movie Home Companion*. New York: Andrews and McMeel.

Ferrara, F. (director). (1979), *Driller Killer*. [film]. Navaron Productions. USA.

Hardy, P. (1986), review in: P. Hardy, T. Milne and P. Willeman (eds.). *Encyclopaedia of Horror Movies*. London: HarperCollins.

Holmes, A. (2002), 'Let There be Blood'. *The Guardian*. July 5 (Review section). 12-3.

Hooper, T. (director). (1976), *Death Trap*. [film]. Mars Production Corporation. USA.

Johnson, L. (director). (1976), *Lipstick*. [film]. De Laurentiis and Paramount Pictures. USA.

Kaplan, J. (director). (1988), *The Accused*. [film]. Paramount Pictures. USA.

Kerekes, D. and D. Slater (2000), *See No Evil: Banned Films and Video*

Controversy. Manchester: Headpress.

Kubrick. S. (director). (1971), *A Clockwork Orange*. [film]. Hawk Films Ltd., Polaris Productions and Warner Bros. UK.
Lehman, P. (1993), 'Don't Blame this on a Girl: Female Rape Revenge Films', in: S. Cohan and I. Hark (eds.). *Screening the Male*. London: Routledge. 103-17.

Lustig, W. (director). (1980), *Maniac*. [film]. Magnum Motion Pictures Inc. USA.

Martin, M. and M. Porter (1991), *Video Movie Guide*. New York: Ballantine.

Newman, K. (1988), *Nightmare Movies*. New York: Harmony.

Mathews, T. (1994), *Censored: The Story of Film Censorship in Britain*. London: Chatto & Windus.

Raimi S. (director). (1982), *The Evil Dead*. [film]. New Line Cinema and Renaissance Pictures. USA.

Starr, Marco (1984), 'J Hills is Alive: A Defence of *I Spit on Your Grave*', in: M. Barker (ed). *The Video Nasties: Freedom and Censorship in the Media*. London: Pluto. 48-55.

Zarchi M. (director). (1978), *I Spit on Your Grave*. [film]. Cinemagic Pictures. USA.

Naked Terror: Horrific, Aesthetic and Healing Images of Rape

Madelaine Hron

How to visually represent the *terror* of rape? How to capture this moment of utter violence - this painful penetration into the most intimate parts of being; this fear, powerlessness and meaninglessness - when one's body, language, personhood and trust in the world are completely lost? How to portray the aggression, brutality and inhumanity of the perpetrator? *Is there* a way to meaningfully represent such violence in our world today, described by some, as a post-traumatic world suffering from compassion fatigue?[1] These are some of the questions that I address in this chapter where I exhibit some publicly-recognizable representations of rape to the privately re-membered artistic creations by rape survivors. A caveat however – this is not the exacting analysis of an historian or a psychotherapist, but rather, the reflections of an observer troubled by this naked terror that casually and even creatively menaces us every day.

Our culture is seemingly suffused with brutal rape images, from graphic rape scenes on such pornography sites coolly called www.rape.to/rape/, or www.rapeandterror.com, rape comics and cartoons in magazines like *Playboy, Hustler* or *Penthouse*, to supposedly realist rape scenes in movies such as *The Accused* and *Boys Don't Cry*.[2] It is beyond the scope of this piece to scrutinize these sights/sites of graphic assault; I find it difficult to analyze them objectively. I allude to them here simply to point out the commercial, entertainment and even pleasure value of rape as a component of consumer culture. I am interested in addressing another type of representation: the *artistic representations of rape* or rape when it is elevated as art. I'll begin by focusing on depictions of rape in *classical art* in order to highlight some of the main themes that render the act into art. I'll then turn to examples of *art therapy* produced by survivors of sexual assault which, as part of the healing process, allows them to express their traumatic memories. My primary question throughout this study, is how to represent rape *aesthetically*; how to make visually palatable such a horrifying event that bears no beauty whatsoever. More importantly, I will ask whether such an act of violence can be represented *at all* via symbol or image, or whether, by the mere act of representation, it necessarily comes to signify something else: an acceptance or legitimization of such violence, or the possibility of healing and transcending it.

1.   Rape in Classical Art

As one surveys celebrated paintings of rape, it is difficult to imagine the terror of sexual assault. Modern images of art especially, attempt to divert and deviate our sensibilities from the dread-filled reality of rape through artsy, creative and innovative approaches. Some paintings seem to make light of the act in a similar way to the *Playboy* and *Penthouse* cartoons. For example, in René Margitte's surrealist depiction *Le Viol (The Rape)* (figure 1), a woman's face/body comes to represent rape. Surrealism claims a mode of art that aims to expose the shadows of the unconscious rather than promote aesthetic principles. In this unconscious vein though, it seems a that unquestionably, a woman's only identity is her body; the implication being she has no mind, no other subjectivity aside from her sex organs. Rape, by extension, is reduced to the objectification of this body - ostensibly, any terror or trauma that rape inflicts on a woman's psyche is expunged. A troubling juxtaposition indeed, albeit amusing to some, because of its black humour perhaps. Similarly perturbing is Christian van Cowenburgh's *Rape of the Negress* (figure 2) where we observe a black woman struggling to escape the clutches of her assailants, while they look on amused: one mockingly points to her distress while the other parodies her helpless gestures. It is an image of warped contempt. Perhaps Cowenburgh is implying the trite banality of this household act, however instead of being convinced by the painting's motives, one can be strangely alienated by it, in much the same shame-filled position as the victim. Images that propose the terror we know we should feel when viewing rape, instead often make us uneasy, as is the case in Pablo Picasso's rendition of the *Rape of the Sabines* (figure 3). The distorted fragmentation of this monochrome aptly captures the confusion and fear residing in the woman whose contorted, bloated body is writhing under the impending phallic hoof of the beast. Yet we also know that Picasso was not particularly kind to his female lovers (two committed suicide while others bore his misogyny, such as Francoise Gilot who writes in her memoirs of the brutal assaults he inflicted upon her). Moreover, contextualizing the work, we realize it is merely a Cubist parody, an abstraction of the classic *Rape of the Sabines*, and thus nothing more than a modern deformation of traditional representations. Given its creative and performative practices, modern art all too often distorts the reality of rape, interpreting it as happenstance or something humorous - certainly not horrific.

Just as the modern paintings above operate to jolt our sensibilities, classical painting serves to cultivate notions of beauty. In so doing, it also functions to develop and reinforce social order. As Diane Wolfthal shows in her brilliant analysis *Images of Rape: The Heroic*

Tradition and Its Alternatives, classic images of rape serve to validate the heroism of the assailant, who as a symbol of authority thus legitimates social violence. Take for example, the classic images of 'The Rape of the Sabines', based on the legend of the Sabine women. This myth refers to the foundation of Rome, in that the children born from this forced collective rape by alien invaders, eventually became the future citizens of Rome. Thus embedded in this depiction is a validation of social violence: despite its brutality, this assault will in the end, create a glorious empire. By its repeated representation, these images of rape continue to reiterate a mythic worldview of justified authoritarian and gendered violence.

Apart from this implied social message, *The Rape of the Sabines* portrated by Poussin, di Giovanni or David, of course also figures as the epitome of classic art aesthetics. As such it seeks to depict beauty and entice the viewer by its visually aesthetic appeal. In so doing, these highly stylized classical versions of the 'Rape of the Sabines' clearly aestheticize and sanitize rape, as in Poussin's version (figure 4). In the Poussin's painting, the women do indeed look distraught, but even in this moment of terror, their hair remains surprisingly in place, and they all manage to maintain an air of nobility and grace. As for their assailants, nothing suggests that they are depraved maniacs or brutal monsters. On the contrary, most of the men, aside from the man wielding a knife in the foreground, display cool and collected (heroic) expressions. Finally, in contrast to the obvious violence in the foreground of the Poussin image, we receive a contradictory message if we direct our gaze towards the centre of the image. There we see a couple walking off leisurely, seemingly absorbed in conversation. Painted in the same blue colour as the vicious struggle in the foreground, this scene is thus linked to the rapes which suggests that in the end, all will be resolved, and eventually the woman will learn to love their assailants. Similar shots of couples strolling along in apparent contentment may be spotted in di Giovanni's representation, which seems even more of a spectacle, as the action occurs in an arena encircled by spectators. Here, aside from the two seized figures on the right hand side, no one seems to be struggling to escape. Rather, everyone appears to passively accept this aggression, and even enjoy watching it.

This sense of passivity and nonchalance links the above images of mass rape, to sites/ sights of individual rape. In Botticelli's *Primavera* for example, we see Zephyrus seize the nymph Chloris: we know from myth that he brutally rapes her, marries her and transforms her into Flora. No one in the image however, appears to notice her predicament. All of these images suggest that gendered violence does not perturb the accepted order of things. This idea   underlies the visual narrative recounted in

Maritini's *Rape of Europa* (figure 5). Here an enclave of women usher Europa off with Jupiter. We then spot her in a stream with a bucking bull longingly looking back at her companions. Finally she is united in rapture with Jupiter: the perfect couple.

Indeed, such passive acceptance of rape may have been the presumed understanding of marriage in the Italian Renaissance when most of these images were commissioned. In his marital treatise *Li Nuptiali* for example, Marc Antonio Alteiri insists that "every nuptial act recalls the rape of the Sabines". He calls the wedding party a "brigata" or raiding party, and points to the fact that the clasping of hands in the marriage ceremony signifies the man showing the woman his right to coerce her with violence.[3] These images then, commissioned by princes, function not only to justify tyrannical terror, but also to elucidate marital doctrine.

Finally, given their aesthetic beauty, classic images of rape aim to seduce the reader, thus appealing to the senses with erotic stimulation. For example, the unveiling of statue Giambognola's *Rape of the Sabine Woman,* inspired a number of published poems, such as one written by Bernardo Davanzati who extolled: "This my Gambondgiola, is your Sabine, for whom you burned with desire."[4] Similarly, the unveiling of Titian's *Rape of Europe* prompted his friend Ludovico Dolce to confess:

> There is no man … so hardened in his being who does
> not feel a warming a softening, a stirring of the blood in
> his veins. It is a real marvel; that if a marble state could
> by the stimuli of its beauty so penetrate the marrow of a
> young man…[5]

If one looks at Giambologna's *Rape of the Sabines,* one is more likely to be drawn to the sinewy beauty of the muscled flesh, than the woman's distraught expression. Similarly, in Titian's or Ruben's *Rape of Europa,* there is only order, lyrical voluptuousness and luxurious beauty. It must also be mentioned, that such artistic depictions of rape permitted a particular erotic pleasure: they allowed the otherwise illicit exposure of female flesh to be exhibited as socially acceptable. In so doing, 'the classic art of rape' allowed men to partake in stimulating voyeuristic pleasure: an indulgence depicted by the curtained man in Titian's *Rape of Lucretia* (figure 6) who is obviously taking as much pleasure in the scene as the rapist.

How then is it possible to depict the terror of rape in art without condemning it as a dreadful, evil act? Wolfthal urges us to consider rape images in Medieval iconography, particularly that of early bibles, where rape is reviled as an immoral and wicked deed. Here rape is stripped of any erotic appeal, and is illustrated in purely descriptive and functional terms so as to illustrate it's illegality and depravity. I find these images particularly useful, both in principle and in practice, to compare with the pictures by survivors today,

These Medieval images in no way portray the rapist as a hero - on the contrary, is presented either as an ordinary person, or as in the case of this gruesome miniature (Figure 7), an *enemy*, a foreign enemy at that: in this instance, the invading Turks. Moreover, in Medieval rape iconography, such as in the pictorial representations of the Biblical stories of the Levite and his wife or the rape of Tamar,[6] the violence of rape is usually recast in a *narrative form* and so described visually as a sequence of events. Though these are well known bible stories (just as in the myths addressed above), the artists felt the need to explain how the rapes came about and what the outcome of these acts may have involved (figure 8). It is as if bible illustrators turned to narrative to somehow rendered this evil act comprehensible as well as reprehensible to the viewer.

It is only in the subtlest details that the actual assault of rape is intimated. Wolfhal points to the fact that usually dishevelled hair or torn clothes signal that a rape has occurred. During the act itself, it is often only a single detail - the man holding the woman by the wrist - which indicates that force was used (figure 9a). As a case in point I offer a comparison between these two bedroom scenes: that of willing partners David and Bathsheba (figure 9b) and the contrasting rape of Tamar (figure 9c): they are different only by a flick of the wrist. Such detailed nuances within the narrative frame, direct us to the difficulty of depicting assault and defining it. This difficulty is portrayed in the Codex Germanicus, an early law code of sorts (figure 10). Though rape here is clearly condemned, the authors have difficulty in describing it adequately. Therein lies the greatest difficulty in depicting rape visually: that of relating the event graphically, yet succinctly, in clear legal terms.

I would also like to add that of all the medieval iconography surveyed in this chapter, the most explicit images were drawn by Catherine de Pisan. She vividly illustrates a rape scene, in a manner that leaves no doubt to its violence and sense of violation. Her drawings (figure 11a-c) are straightforward, blunt caricatures, yet it is obvious that the sexual exchange is unsolicited aggression: the woman is clearly the victim, but also a subject, who is refusing male advances.

2.   Contemporary Images of Rape
It was not until the 20th century with the work of feminists such as Nicole Eisenman and Susan Coe, that rape was graphically depicted, so as to

leave no question in the viewers' mind as to the immoral and horrific nature of the act. Susan Coe's *New Bedford Rape* (figure 12) is a rough, shadowy, dark sketch of gang rape. When I saw this image for the first time, after gradually adjusting my eyes to its indistinct obscurity, I realized that the focal point was a woman's body drawn out in sinewy contracted muscles. I quickly averted my eyes and dared not look back.

The question that assailed me when I first approached the art, created by a local group of women survivors of sexual assault in the Detroit region, was – how can one visually respond to or even describe such an ineffable event? I first encountered this type of art at an awareness-raising campaign at my university, The University of Michigan, Ann Arbor. I was inspired, impressed and intrigued, and so became involved with the Washtenaw Sexual Crisis Centre where I later interviewed some artist-survivors about their artwork. Through this exchange I began to understand much more about the struggles and successes of this form of art therapy.

Just as high art advanced the heroism, humour or horror of rape - these images differ drastically in their aim: they seek *to heal* survivors of such horror. This therapeutic technique was developed by psychotherapists to aid traumatized patients in expressing their pain and trying to come to terms with their disjointed world. Such suffering can often not be conveyed in words, but in this practice it is recreated and symbolized anew, in artistic form.

Debates arise as to *whether such pain can be signified in words or symbols.* Leading pain theorist Elaine Scarry argues that pain, particularly excessive pain, is inexpressible, in that the event of pain inevitably destroys language itself: "Its resistance to language is not simply one of those incidental or accidental attributes, but it is essential to what it is."[7] Others such as Wittgenstein claim that there is no such pre-linguistic, private language, even in the subjective experience of pain. They theorize that all language is communicable to others via a certain code. Nietzsche, his *Genealogy of Morals,* proposes that pain is in fact the 'mnemotechnics' by which the social order is constituted and authorized:

> How to create a memory for the human animal? ... 'If something is to stay in the memory it must be burned in: only that which never ceases to hurt stays in our memory.'- this is the main clause of the oldest (unhappily the most enduring) psychology on earth ... [8]

In *Birth of Tragedy* however, Nietzsche develops "the remedy of art" in which aesthetics would prove the means of transcending this social order:

"Art is therapeutic and the artist is a healer who overcomes alienation and depletion to create works that return power and the will to live to individuals living in a decaying, barbaric, and spiritually-bereft culture."[9] To what extent might such art be "a remedy" for these survivors? In *Suffering and The Remedy of Art*, Schweitzer, following Nietzsche, argues that art is perhaps the only means of expressing such pain, in that both pain and art are untranslatable and pre-symbolic. Likewise Scarry, who at first theorizes the "pre-representational" and "prelinguistic nature of pain", focuses, in the second half of her book, on the "re-creation of the world": how subjects in pain grant meaning to their experience, through art or "meaningful artifact" in which they recreate their world. Art therapy grants survivors a different means of expressing their unspeakable pain that does not rely on language, words and narrative. It offers the possibility for meaning through a singular artifact.

Art therapy presents a distinctive quality which traditional narrative psychotherapy does not: the possibility of creation. As the Standing Committee for the Art Therapies Professions explains: "The aim of the sessions is to provide a symbolic language which can provide access to unacknowledged feelings and a means of integrating them creatively into the personality, in order that therapeutic change may take place." The creative act grants the patient a different type of power than traditional narrative therapy can: the opportunity to invent and take mastery over their emotions in an act of self-healing.[10] The therapist doesn't focus on the artistic merit of the work, but on the therapeutic process, that is, on the patients' involvement with their work, their perception of it and the relationship between their art and their traumatic experience.

The images under analysis here were displayed at the *Creative Expressions Exhibit*, sponsored by the Southeast Michigan Anti-Rape Network in the Detroit Public Library from April 4th - May 4th, 2002. The primary aim of this exhibition was to raise awareness about rape and sexual assault. This work clearly represents imagery that the artists wanted to publicly expose. Each piece was produced individually and willingly outside structured art therapy sessions, I do not however, know to what extent it was used in therapy. The survivors explained that the primary purpose of their highly personal work, was to facilitate healing and catharsis: they simply chose to draw, paint or show something about their experience. As they did this they reflected on how their memories and feelings changed in the process of rendering rape into art. As one of the artists put it, they aimed to *"make some sense out of all the fear"* and *"make something beautiful out of all that horror."* As art therapist Louis Thomas argues, art therapy "re-presentation" or "the concrete evocation of trauma through art-making" is different from artistic representation in that, instead of standing in or symbolizing an event, it "embodies the feelings of abuse in a concrete form rather than expressing its contents symbolically or metaphorically."[11] Yet, despite Thomas' contention and the artists' intentions, I was profoundly surprised and even staggered by the meaningfulness of the art displayed.

As I pored over these images, the first thing that struck me was the amount of effort that had gone into showing something meaningful, but above all *understandable*, in each piece. Like Medieval iconography, these images all reveal the difficulty of representing rape and the feelings attached to being raped, in a symbolic form that can be clearly understood by the viewer. It is almost as if they were attempting to identify the terror and pain they felt, and continue to feel, while at the same time trying to *convince* the viewer of its absolute reality. In this way, the images remind me of Scarry's statement, "To be in great pain is to have certainty, to hear of great pain is to have doubt."[12]

Much of the artwork displayed at the Detroit exhibit were poster collages, with words and images cut out from newspapers and magazines. By recycling media clippings in this way, survivors were able to verbalize their feelings with simple referents and name the manifold, often conflicting emotions, that overwhelm them without having to visually depict such complex feelings. Many art therapy self-help books encourage this type of poster-work in order to help survivors find the words and images they are missing, to express their experience.[13] The collage titled *Shame* for example, offers multiple shades of self-contemptuous feelings through synonyms like "little" "gone" "ugly" "monster" "nothing," "empty," "horrible" "it". This kind of articulation urges viewers to think about the feelings and thoughts associated with the 'shame' felt by many survivors.

Some of these collage posters proffered powerful social commentary, especially *Forget-me not* (figure 13). It was this collage that inspired me to take up this project of contrasting classical and art therapy pictures. The simple poster features a flower composed of classical rape paintings ranging from Rueben's *Rape of Europa* and Poussin's *Rape of the Sabines* to modern works such as Mull's radical *Oh Sensibility* (which photographs a contorted man with a duck on his head astride a naked woman) and Ana Mendiata's rape performance-documentary *Rape-Murder* (featuring a bloodied body abandoned among the leaves). This aesthetic flower is rained upon by rain from a nebulous cloud titled "virtual rape". The caustic rain drops down such unbelievable newspaper headings as "Is Rape a Symbol?," "Is Rape a War of the Sexes" "Rape - A Tactic In The War Of The Sexes." Before reaching the ground, the titles condense into headlines of actual rapes, murders, legal decrees, and statistics, such as that one third of women will be raped in their life-time or that battery is the most unreported crime in US. The sun shining on this merry scene (figure 13b) brightly heralds to "expect more pillage and rape as men become the new oppressed" while its rays burst forth toddler incest or infant and baby gang-rapes. Clearly, this poster purposefully reappropriates stereotypical images of erotic paintings in counterpoint with ludicrous and sensationalist newspaper headings, in order to show how these all construct "virtual rape", which, like a bright sunny day, allows us to forget the reality of rape.

Among the art, there were also two very poignant series, which intimately and explicitly depict rape. As I am told, they are not representative of the 'real' rapes that these individuals endured - rather they are abstractions or analogous representations. As one survivor put it, "We are not artists, we don't really have the skills or the strength to draw what really happened. Or to draw our abuser - God no! We just try to make images. We somehow make sense of what happened to us and how we feel about it."

The first arduous attempt to capture the terror of rape is a set of sketches, which traumatically repeats the same scene over and over again – that of the assailant entering a bedroom – obviously a moment of great fear and terror for the artist as she draws it again and again, refining it every time. In her detailed review of trauma, Judith Herman writes of the "omnipresent fear of death" and "overwhelming sense of helplessness"[14] experienced by the abused child: such signs of trauma are clearly evident here, in these images of hypervigilence, or 'frozen watchfulness.' The first picture of the sequence (14a) is drawn quickly and crudely, with the pencil heavily shadowing in a figure in a doorway, almost as if the artist is desperately trying to get it out; to hastily put the scene on paper. In the second attempt (14b) there is obvious anger as a male form, cast roughly into the paper, emerges from the previous shadow, taking up almost the whole doorway. The horizontal lines intimate that something lies beyond the frame. The third sketch (14c) contrasts with the previous two. In a more delicate effort to outline the situation, the pencil sketches the man in fine spindly lines. In the original there is evidence of much erasing, obviously the artist was trying to get the muscles and body structure just right. In this respect this image looks almost aesthetic and even erotic, as beyond the door we see the body of a woman. The final image (14d) differs markedly from the previous one: the artist reverts to the heavy shadowing and contouring, emphasizing the darkness of the bedroom and thus the terror of the scene. As for the shape of the man, it is certainly not beautiful but monstrous; his flesh is sinewy; he is weirdly contorted and marked up, and the shape of his head indicates a sense of the bestial. This is the first time we see the assailant moving stealthily and, also the first time we see his hands, which appear to have claws. We clearly identify the shape of a woman, her head turned away as if sleeping. These examples show the complexity of portraying a prelude to rape through the ordinary action of a man entering a bedroom. *Not only must the survivor define what is happening, but she must move beyond conventional norms of male beauty and heroism* to fully seize the dread that accompanies this event.

The previous example also shows a turn towards *a narrative and thematic structure*, as in the Biblical iconography. This narrative turn becomes unmistakable in the next series of paintings - the most explicit sequence of all, and for me, the most disturbing. We see the fragment of a woman as a white unmarked hand opens a door. We then see the same erased body-build atop a woman in various positions - the colour in the background becoming progressively more ominous (figure 15a-c). The most graphic image is the magenta red spectre-shape between her taut outstretched and bruised legs (figure 15b). Here the assailant is completely whited-out and literally burns into the background behind him, as if the artist poured some paint thinner or acid onto his form to make any trace of him completely vanish. The final tableau (figure 15c) shows the woman completely crouched over, in utter contrast to the first image (15a) where she is sitting upright. Here her bloated, bruised form resembles a bleeding uterus.

What is particularly perturbing about this image, and even the preceding one, is *the overwhelming and overpowering position of the assailant-rapist* - the terror that bears no name, and thus cannot be symbolized. In the sketches, the man takes up the whole door-frame, and here the blanked-out body overwhelms almost the entire image. The importance of the rapist is made even more explicit in *The Rapists* (figure 16). This poster displays some fifty pictures of men and women, almost as a family album. Only the blood smeared on the sides gives it away as of prisoners holding up ID plaques or being measured. The work is actually composed of mug-shots taken from internet lists of US Convicted Rapists and US Most Wanted Sex Offenders. I do not know what could possibly prompt a survivor to seek out, browse through, cut and paste photos of rapists for display, yet this act obviously offered her some form of healing. Perhaps, much like her perpetrator she had to find her 'victims', expose them and shame them in this act. Her action may also serve as a public service warning. I subsequently learned she also composed another collage based on sex offender lists, titled *128 Among You,* the number of perpetrators still at large in her county.

Clearly, such a fixated focus on the aggressor deflects attention from the victim, and *puts into question the subjectivity of the victim-*

survivor. In the previous images the woman's body is seems to be missing, fragmented, severed or blocked out, by the rapist or media clippings. This therapeutic art-work therefore, differs most radically from classical representations of pain in art, (as highlighted for example in *Iconographia del Dolore, Torment in Art* or *Pictures of the Body: Pain and Metamorphosis*.) Here the primary means of conveying pain is through of the human form. In renowned paintings by Picasso, Munch, Van Gogh, pain is conveyed by means of the flesh, most notably in the contorted, sinewy and grimacing expressions of an open mouth and supplicating eyes. Medieval representations of torture scenes and executions in *Torment in Art*, clearly show two types of victims, the innocent and the guilty. The dichotomy is marked by their eyes, either harsh or beseeching, and their body, either indefinite (the guilty) or painstakingly detailed and writhing in torment (the innocent). When we compare these to the art therapy images, there is no comparison: the guilty ones seem to be the victims - their bodies either missing or mere forms.

The representation of the human form suggests agency, identity and selfhood. In social discourse, individuality and identity also generates a meaningful response from the public. In the case of rape, most literature on sexual abuse supports the notion that regaining a sense of self, a love of one's body, a feeling of safety in the world, and power and control stemming from one's personal abilities, is the greatest challenge for survivors. During a rape, the victim is completely helpless, his/her body is snatched from her/him, and his/her sense of safety and trust in the world is irrevocably shattered. For this reason, these last images are perhaps the most poignant: they suggest a return to the self in an attempt to regain a sense of identity.

The final set of images aims to *reclaim and rescue the human subject* by reconstructing the survivors' bodies and, most notably, their *voice*. Among these corporeal images, is a painting of a female body, albeit partial and fragmented, which reveals the delicate folds of the body self. Painted in soft hues, this oil painting (figure 17) displays the sensuous stomach of a woman curled in the vulnerable foetus position. Contrasting this image is a rather rough painting of woman's hands crossed over her chest, either in shame or in defiance (figure 18). Finally there is a large painting, *Scream!* painted in with firm and thick brush strokes in a vivid red and black (figure 19). The explanation attached to the painting states the following: "What my heart wants to do, but cannot." These last images are able to draw us into the body-self inscribed through rape. As such, they are as powerfully affective as the classical images that seek to seduce us with erotic appeal. The crucial difference in the contemporary art- therapy work, is that the spectator is more likely to be moved to sympathy and empathize with the survivors' trauma, shame and loss.

Despite their therapeutic intent, many of the healing images are not mere therapy: they are art in themselves. I would like to conclude with a piece titled *Always On My Mind* (figure 20). In many ways it differs from the other representations, in that it is more metaphorical and abstract, and is able to return us to the earlier modern art images addressed in this essay. At first, we see what appears to be a brain scan. Upon a closer inspection though, it explodes as a clear and explicit representation of the ineffable terror of rape that has been indelibly impressed upon the survivor's mind as monument and memory.

Rape is terrible, terror-able evil indeed. It en-ables terror -- in the acutely agonizing act itself, but perhaps also, more subtly and perniciously, in the act of representation as well. As we have seen in these varied images, representations of rape can be actual or aesthetic, rendering rape accessible or distancing it, serving to heal this evil or perpetrate it. I hope that this chapter inspires many questions about the nature of art and the nature of evil, but above all, I hope that it allows us to draw the intimate relationship between the two. Can art really express the terror of rape? In the presence of such evil, should art speak? Then again, in the face of such cruelty, can art ever be silent? It is up to us, witnesses to evils, to recognize the representations that enable us and those that terrorize us. Either to consider all art, be it classical, contemporary and therapy-based, as virtual 'forget-me-nots.' Or to keep these imprints 'always on our minds,' as testaments to the naked terror of rape.

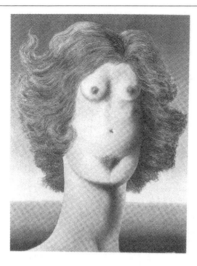

Figure 1. René Magritte (1934), *Le viol* (The Rape)
© C. Herscovici, Brussels/Artists Right Society (ARS), New York.

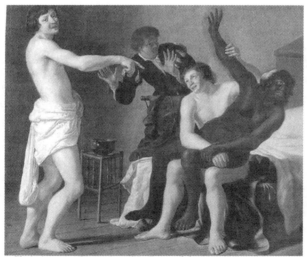

Christian van Cowenburgh's *Rape of the Negress*

Figure 2. Cowenburg (1632) *Rape of Negress*. Musee des Beaux Arts.
Strasbourg

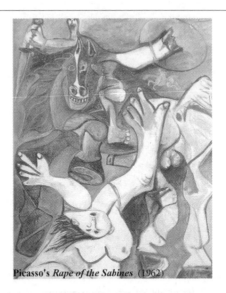

Figure 3. Picasso (1962), *Rape of the Sabines*. © 2002 Museum of Fine Arts. Boston

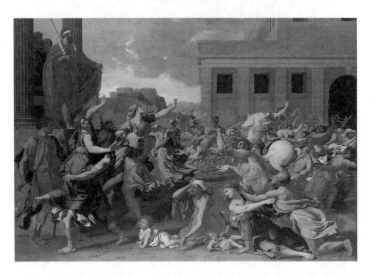

Figure 4. Poussin (1636-7), *Rape of the Sabine Women*. Metropolitan Museum of Art. New York (Harris Brisbane Dick Fund, 1941. 41. 160)

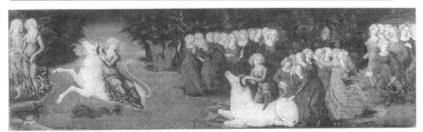

Francesco di Giorgio Martini's *Rape of Europa* |

Figure 5. Francisco Martini (c.1500), *Rape of the Sabines*, Musee du
Louvre. Paris.

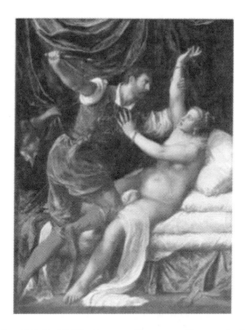

Figure 6. Titian (1559-1962), *Rape of Lucretia*. Boston Isabella Stewart
Gardner Museum. Boston.

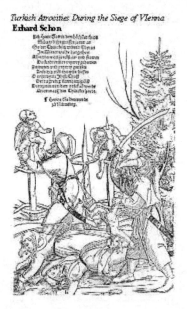

Figure 7. Erhard Schon. *Turkish Atrocities during the Siege of Vienna.*
location unknown.

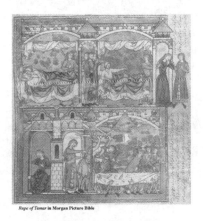

Figure 8. *David and Bathsheba.* (detail) Morgan Picture Bible ca. 1240 –
55. The Pierpoint Morgan Library. M638 fol 41v. New York.

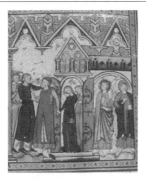

9a. (ca. 1240-55), *Rape of Dinah,* Plate 3b.23 (detail) Morgan Picture Bible. Reprint Cambridge England by W.Lewis 1927.

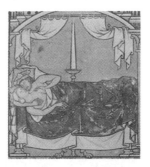

Figure 9b. Ibid. *David and Batsheba.*

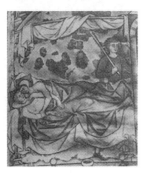

Figure 9c. Ibid., *Rape of Tamar.*

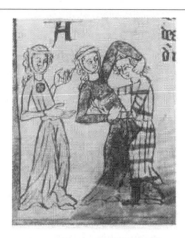

Figure 10. (shortly before 1315), *Rape of an "Amie" Sachenspiel*. Codex Palatinus Germanicus. 164, fol. 20. Heidelberg Universitats bibliothek.

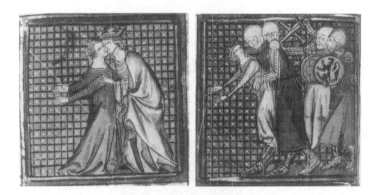

Figure 11a and b. Pisan (ca 1325-50), *Boreas and Oreithia Ovide moralise*. MS5069. fol.92. Bibliotheque de l'arsenal. Paris. *Paris et Helen*. idem fol. 162.

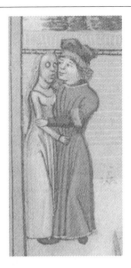

Figure 11c. Pisan. (1904), *Pigmalion dans son Atelier* Plate 22, 25v from *Epistle from Othea to Hector*. Reproduction. London: J.B Nichols.

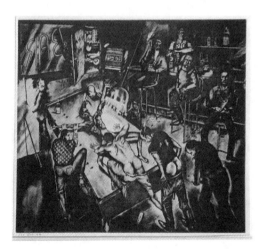

Figure 12. Coe. *New Bedford Rape*. St. Etienne Gallery. New York

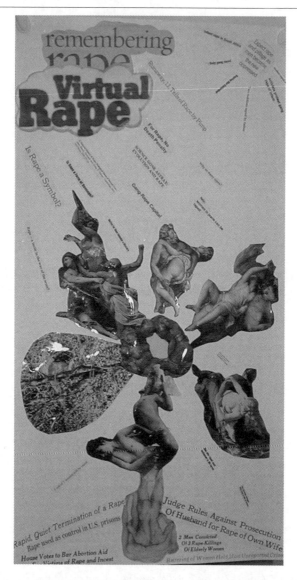

Figure 13a. Anonymous (2002), 'Creative Expressions Exhibit',
sponsored by the Southeast Michigan Anti-Rape Network. Detroit Public
Library

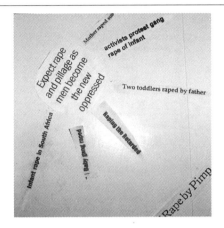

Figure 13b. Ibid.

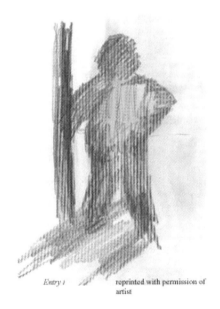

Figure 14a. Ibid.

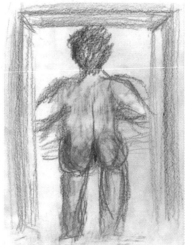

The Entry (ii)   reprinted with permission of artist

Figure 14b. Ibid

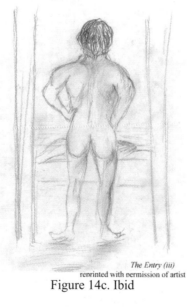

The Entry (iii)
reprinted with permission of artist

Figure 14c. Ibid

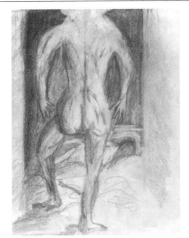

The Entry (IV) --reprinted with permission of artist

Figure 14d. Ibid.

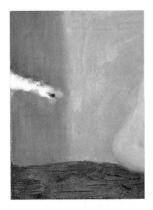

Figure 15a. Ibid

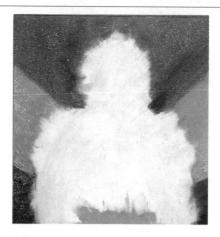

Figure 15b. Ibid

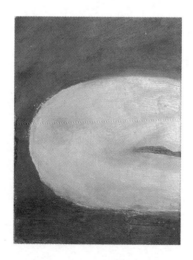

Figure 15c. Ibid.

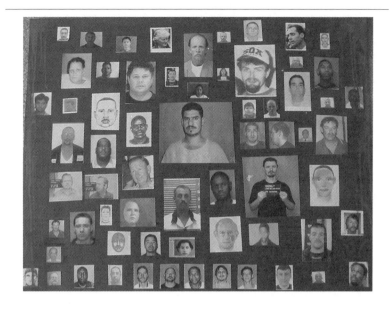

Figure 16. Ibid.

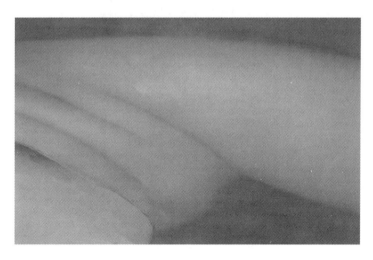

Figure 17. Ibid.

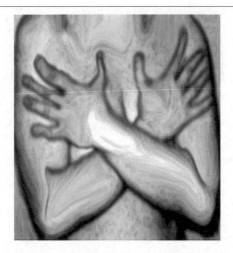

.Figure 18. Ibid.

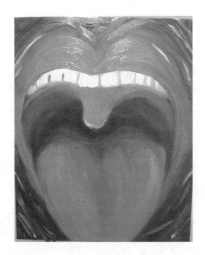

Figure 19. Ibid.

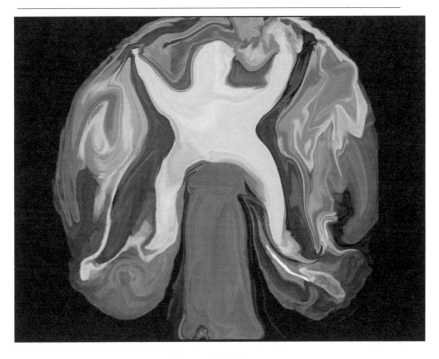

Figure 20. Ibid.

Notes

1. Farrell 1998 and Moeller, 1999.
2. For examples see: http://www.oneangrygirl.net/wackyrape.html.
3. Witthoft, 1982, 47.
4. Heikamp, 1989, 55.
5. Ginzburg,1989,81-2.
6. Judges 19; 2 Samuel 13.
7. Scarry, 1989, 5.
8. Nietzsche, 1996, 60-61.
9. Nietzsche, 1956, xiv.
10. Therapists such as Jennings (1996) would argue that creative therapies such as art therapy, play therapy or dramatherapy, are in fact better than traditional psychotherapy which "often robs the person of their own power and self-healing capacity" (202) as well as creating unequal roles between the therapist and client.
11. Thomas, 1998, 29.
12. Scarry, 7.
13. See Cappacchione, 1990; Mines, 1996; Davis, 1990 or Allender, 1995, 41.
14. Herman, 1992, 98.

References

Allender, D. (1995), *The Wounded Heart: Hope for Adult Victims of Childhood Sexual Abuse*, Colorado Springs: NavPress.

Capacchione, L. (1990) *The Picture of Health: Healing Your Life With Art,* Santa Monica, Calif: Hay House.

Davis, L. (1990). *The Courage to heal workbook : for women and men survivors of child sexual abuse.* New York, N.Y.: Harper & Row.

Elkins, J.(1999), *Pictures of the Body : Pain and Metamorphosis.* Stanford, Calif.: Stanford University Press.

Farrell, K. (1998), *Post-Traumatic Culture : Injury and Interpretation in the Nineties.* Baltimore: Johns Hopkins University Press.

Finizio, G, and Accademia di belle arti (Milan Italy). (1994) *Iconografia Del Dolore.* Milano: Electa.

Gilot, F. and C. Lake (1964*), Life with Picasso*. New York: McGraw-Hill.

Ginzburg, C. (1989), *Clues Myths and the Historical Method.* (trans.) J. and A Tedeschi. Baltimore London: John Hopkins University Press.

Heikamp, D. (1989) "A Rare Booklet of Poems on Giambologna's Rape of a Sabine Woman," *Paragone,* 40 (November 1989): 52-70.

Herman, J. L. (1992). *Trauma and recovery.* New York, N.Y.: BasicBooks.

Jennings, S. (1996), 'Brief Dramatherapy: The healing power of the dramatized here and now', in: A. Gersie (ed) *Dramatic Approaches to Brief Therapy.* London: Jessica Kingsley.

Kaplan, J. (director) (1988), *The Accused.* [film]. Paramount Pictures. USA

Mines, S. (1996) *Sexual Abuse/Sacred Wound: Transforming Deep Trauma,* Barrytown NY: Barrytown Ltd..

Moeller, S. D. (1999), *Compassion Fatigue : How the Media Sell Disease, Famine, War, and Death.* New York: Routledge.

Nietzsche, F. W., D. Smith, et al. (1996), *On the genealogy of morals :a polemic : by way of clarification and supplement to my last book, Beyond good and evil.* Oxford: Oxford University Press.

Nietzsche, F. W. (1956), *The birth of tragedy and The genealogy of morals.* Garden City, N.Y.: Doubleday.

Peirce, K. (director) (1999), *Boy's Don't Cry.* [film]. Hart-Sharp Entertainment, Independent Film Channel, Killer Films. USA.

Puppi, L.(1991) *Torment in Art : Pain, Violence, and Martyrdom.* New York: Rizzoli.

Scarry, E. (1985), *The body in pain : the making and unmaking of the world.* New York: Oxford University Press.

Schweizer, H. (1997), *Suffering and the Remedy of Art.* Albany: State University of New York Press.

Te Paske, B. A. (1982). *Rape and ritual : a psychological study*. Toronto: Inner City Books.

Thomas, L, (1998) 'Re-Presentation To Representations of Sexual Abuse', in: D. Sandle (ed) *Development and diversity : new applications in art therapy*. New York: Free Association Books. p. 29-40.

Witthoft, B. (1982) 'Marriage Rituals and Marriage Chests in Quattrocento Florence'. *Artibus et Historiae*. 5: 43-59.

Wolfthal, D. (1999), *Images of rape: the "heroic" tradition and its alternatives*. New York: Cambridge University Press.

––––

This paper would not have been possible without the help of many people. I would thank all the artist survivors who shared their experience with me, but above all, I would like to thank Linden Thoburn from the *Washtenaw Sexual Assault Crisis Centre* whose support enabled me to undertake and complete this project.

Part III

Crime: Versions of Guilt, Shame and Redemption

Masking the Evil of Capital Punishment[*]

Earl F. Martin

The evil that men do lives after them;
The good is oft interred with their bones.

Shakespeare, Julius Caesar act 3, sc. 2.

In light of the fact that the subject matter of this chapter is capital punishment, it's probably not surprising to find that the title includes the word evil and starts out with a quote speaking to the impact of evil on the world. After all, it has, or at least almost has, become a cliché to refer to our death row inmates and their heinous crimes as prime examples of the existence of evil in our time. This chapter's concern with the tie that binds evil and capital punishment however, will not focus on the crimes that place men on death row. Instead, the 'evil that men do' under consideration in these pages, is the evil that the state embraces when it deliberately puts a condemned inmate to death.

Inherent within the previous paragraph is the assertion that the infliction of the death penalty upon another is an act of evil and this is a proposition that will undoubtedly invite challenge from some quarters. The claim that capital punishment is evil is based on the fact that state-sponsored killings do not serve the interests of deterrence or retribution, the two principles of punishment that are put forward as justifying the sanction's use. This makes an execution the unjustified intentional killing of another, and thus, injurious to society's collective moral or physical happiness or welfare. This means that executions are evil.

The long running debate over deterrence and capital punishment, has arrived at the point where the weight of the considered opinion across the spectrum of the general public to criminal justice experts, is that the death penalty offers no statistically significant deterrent benefit beyond that offered by long-term confinement.[1] Therefore, death penalty supporters have been left to advance an intuition based claim, in favour of deterrence, which asserts that there are obviously some individuals who are contemplating murder and will decide not to do so, because if they are caught and convicted they may very well be executed, and death is a natural human fear.[2] This intuition based claim however, is far removed from a true inquiry into whether the death penalty is justified. If we are

---

[*] A version of this chapter appears in volume 10.2 of the *Virginia Journal of Social Policy & the Law*

searching for affirmative proof that the death penalty accomplishes an accepted purpose of criminal punishment, as we should be, the record on deterrence is lacking to the point of non-existence. In effect, the intuition grounded argument is one that says we should continue to execute murderers because we have always executed murderers. It was just this sort of logic that U.S. Supreme Court Justice Oliver Wendell Holmes had in mind when he wrote, "It is revolting to have no better reason for a rule of law than that so it was laid down in the time of Henry IV."[3]

As for retribution serving as a justifying principle for capital punishment, whatever appeal retribution might have in a world with a just death penalty system, that appeal quickly fades in the face of how the sanction is carried out in the United States.[4] This argument rests on the fact that our capital punishment system generates unprincipled death sentences because of the influence that certain institutional infirmities exert on the outcome of individual cases. Although not an exclusive list of the problems that arguably plague the administration of our death penalty, the incompetence of defense counsel,[5] the influence of racial bias,[6] and the wrongful conviction and execution of the innocent[7] serve as prime examples for how the real life of our death penalty undercuts its theoretical retributive underpinnings. The death penalty that is employed in the United States - which works from the premise that executions should be reserved for only the worst offenders - is one that instead ends up being, "haphazardly administered against a small, almost randomly selected sample of eligible persons."[8] As a consequence, the moral force that is supposed to underlie a legitimate search for retribution is radically undercut by the true nature of our system, which results in many of the condemned who enter our execution chambers, being given a death that they did not, under any circumstances, deserve.

The assertion that the infliction of the death penalty upon another is an act of evil raises a very significant question. Namely, if capital punishment is evil, why is it that the sanction is so widely embraced in the United States? In other words, how can it be that thirty-eight American states and the U.S. federal government all approve of a form of criminal punishment that is purported to be an evil practice? Providing at least a partial answer to the central question just posed will be the focus of the main body of this chapter.

1.   Masking the Evil

Although the following is not the sole explanation for why the evil practice of capital punishment continues to thrive across the United States, one core reason for this state-of-affairs is that Americans, of which the author is one, have done a very effective job of shielding themselves from the critical nature of the death penalty. That is, in a number of different ways, the ultimate fact of the death penalty - that we are killing our fellow human beings - is masked by the process that surrounds the event.

The most obvious example of an evil masking phenomenon within America's capital punishment system, is that executions take place behind prison walls and locked doors, so that the public do not have to witness these spectacles. Removing executions from the public view creates the tendency for the sanction to fall into the 'out of sight, out of mind' category of events, which, in turn, encourages us to avoid confronting the moral consequences of our actions.

In addition to the explicit removal of executions from the public square, we employ more subtle means by which we hide the evil of capital punishment from ourselves in an effort to salve our collective conscience. Through the bureaucratization of executions, the inclusion of lawyers and medical doctors within the system, and the employment of religious themes and activities in connection with the sanction, we manage to push the evil that is inherent in capital punishment either out of view or, at least, to a place of minor significance in weighing the pros and cons of the sanction.

In carrying out a modern day execution, very little is left to chance by the bureaucrats in charge. Every step of the process is managed and each participant's role is scripted, with the result being that personal responsibility is minimized and real-life human reactions are suppressed.[9] For example, in Washington State there is a manual that details exactly what kind of rope is to be used and how it is to be prepared for those condemned men who chose hanging over lethal injection.[10] An ex-warden of the Mississippi State Penitentiary has described how green clip-on cards were issued to execution team members while official witnesses got yellow cards, and how his staff practiced upcoming executions, complete with a stand-in that would be strapped into the gas chamber chair and hooked-up to an EKG monitor.[11] In Texas, the bureaucratic preparation for death begins about two weeks before the execution, and covers such items as selecting witnesses for the event, securing telephone contact with the governor's office, and notifying a local funeral home to make arrangements for removal of the inmate's body.[12] In Utah, depending on whether the method of execution is by firing squad or lethal injection, one member of the execution team is assured of either firing a blank or releasing a harmless solution, so that no one knows who actually caused the prisoner's death.[13]

The net effect of this bureaucratization of executions, is to present them as clinical and controlled events, which in turn allows a sense of mundanity to settle on the state killing its own. One commentator has written that the procedures, "smack of a mechanized, mindless nihilism"[14] in recognition of the fact that the process allows everyone within the system, from the clerk who inventories the condemned prisoner's worldly possessions to the executioner who starts the toxic mix of drugs flowing into the prisoner's veins to say, "I'm only doing my job. I didn't kill him." Thereafter, when the rest of us learn of the execution through media reports, and absorb such trivia as the amount of time the prisoner spent with his family or what he ate for his last meal, we are encouraged to similarly bury our heads in the sand. Instead of thinking of ourselves as the prisoner's collective executioner, we find comfort in the belief that the killing we read about in our morning paper was not the result of our efforts, but rather the work of some omnipotent process far removed from our realm of responsibility.

Like the near-clandestine nature of state executions and the overall bureaucratization of the process, the role of the lawyers and doctors in our system of capital punishment contributes mightily to the ability of the sanction to hide behind a patina of legitimacy. Notwithstanding image problems that plague these professions from time-to-time, our opinion leaders are often attorneys and doctors. The participation of these men and women throughout the death penalty chain gives us the peace of mind that our best and brightest are in charge, so everything must be okay.

Because the American system of capital punishment purports to be grounded in the rule of law, lawyers are distributed throughout that system. A large number of the legislators and executives who champion death penalty statutes are lawyers, and many of these are not shy about letting the public know that they believe the death penalty is a necessary and appropriate punishment for serious crime.[14] Furthermore, all of the judges who preside over death penalty cases at trial and hear these cases on appeal are lawyers. In fulfilling their duties, these professionals convey to the public the impression that the system is stable and working properly. Moreover, beyond sending this far-reaching message, trial and appellate judges more immediately enable capital sentencing jurors to avoid confronting the full impact of what it means to condemn another human being to death.

When trial judges preside over a capital case in accordance with the accepted legal rules and procedures, they, at least implicitly, convey a message to the jurors that death is the lawfully preferred sanction and that the jurors should not feel personally responsible for selecting that result. First, by administering and enforcing the death-qualifying procedures that are employed in the selection of capital jurors which exclude citizens who oppose the death penalty, trial judges may send the message that the legitimate and favoured position in the legal system is one supporting death.[16] This message, in turn, may lead capital jurors to believe they are personally obligated and legally bound to 'follow the law' by choosing capital punishment over available alternatives. Second, by adhering to the dominate restrictive view of what constitutes mitigating evidence, trial judges deny the defense the opportunity to impress upon the jurors the full weight of the moral decision that confronts them. By not allowing capital sentencing jurors to hear about the despair and stress of life on death row, the impact that state-sponsored executions have on the lives of condemned men's families, and the horrors of the executions themselves, trial judges prevent jurors from having the information they need to fully understand and appreciate the consequences of their decision.[17] Third, the confusing and complicated sentencing instructions that are part of a capital case have a tendency to encourage jurors to see their role as one of applying a legal formula instead of rendering a moral decision. As one commentator on our criminal justice system has put it, "these badly framed and poorly understood instructions seem to provide jurors with a protective shield that enables them to avoid a sense of personal responsibility for their decisions ..."[18]

In addition to contributing to our collective ease towards capital punishment by providing additional levels of review for death penalty cases, appellate judges also provide 'cover' for capital sentencing jurors when they are required to chose between life and death. Believing that others up the line will subject their verdict to a searching review allows jurors to, "distance themselves from the moral implications of ... [their] awesome responsibility by maintaining the belief that someone else - typically appellate judges - will ultimately decide [the defendant's fate]."[19] Paradoxically, "the very judges on whom capital jurors rely to review and 'correct' their decisions also defer to and rely on the jury's decision to insulate themselves from the moral issues posed by death verdicts."[20] In the end though, the interplay in capital cases between jurors, trial judges and appellate judges, gives the appearance of a system that squarely faces the gravity of its task: the diffusion of responsibility between these actors enables them to avoid having to fully experience the monumental decision to kill another human being.

At the level of the litigants in a capital case, the prosecutors who seek and secure the death penalty for defendants and who frequently speak publicly in favour of the sanction, are all lawyers. Through their actions and words, these opinion leaders allow us to rest assured that trusted public officials are making sure that only the 'right' defendants are being put at risk of death. Additionally, at trial these attorneys, consistent with the dominant paradigm that focuses on weapons and wounds, instrumentalities and effects, employ legal rules and procedures to present the defendant as nothing more than the heinous crime that has brought him into the courtroom facing the prospect of the ultimate sanction. By doing so, prosecutors contribute mightily to the ability of capital jurors and the public at large to disengage from the accused and come to see him as something *other*. Once this view is established, feelings of empathy for the accused are highly unlikely, thus lessening the jurors' burden in choosing death over life, and the public's burden in supporting that choice.[21]

Like the prosecutors who champion the case for death, except in those rare instances of a pro se defendant, all of those who advocate in court against the imposition of the sanction in specific cases, are lawyers. To the extent that these attorneys, for whatever reason, fail to present a mitigation case in sentencing, they, like the prosecutors who demonize the defendant, make it easier for a juror to morally disengage from the defendant's humanity and render a verdict for death. Furthermore, while the efforts of defense attorneys do not offer an endorsement for capital punishment, those efforts do contribute to the sanction's patina of legitimacy, just as do the efforts of legally trained legislators, executives, judges, and prosecutors. Because defense counsel are cast in the role of keeping the system honest and faithful, they add to the ability of the system to maintain its respectability as it moves men along to their deaths.[22]

The two most controversial ways that doctors participate in the American system of capital punishment are in the treatment of the insane condemned and by participating in executions.[23] As for the first instance, the Supreme Court has held that the Eighth Amendment prohibits the death penalty from being carried out upon a prisoner who is insane.[24] Therefore, before the state can execute a condemned man that has lapsed into insanity, it must make him sane: this means employing medical professionals to cure the mental affliction, if they can. Insanity issues aside, when a condemned prisoner enters the death chamber to be executed, a medical professional will frequently be on hand to pronounce the prisoner dead and certify the time of death, and, in some jurisdictions, may even directly participate in the actual execution. Curing the insane condemned and attending or participating in executions, has caused great controversy within the medical profession, but it is not the purpose of this work to comment on the specifics of those debates. Rather, the involvement of doctors in support of the capital punishment system is mentioned because it, like the actions of lawyers within that process, sends a message to the public that all is well. Curing the insane, placing a catheter in a man's vein, and/or leaning over a corpse to check for a pulse, are actions that allow executions to take on the appearance of being something similar to a medical procedure. In other words, the presence of these medical professionals lures us into believing that what is unfolding in our death chambers, is an everyday medical event as opposed to an act of evil in which the state deliberately takes the life of another.

The removal of executions from public view and the bureaucratization of the process that surrounds these killings, both tend to obscure the evil that lurks beneath the sanction by lessening the moral impact of the final event. Likewise, the role of doctors and lawyers in the administration of the death penalty tends to allow state-sanctioned executions to hide behind a curtain of respectability that is constructed out of the function that these professionals serve within society. The last evil masking phenomenon to be taken up here is arguably the most pervasive of all, because it is arguably one of the most pervasive phenomenon in all walks of life. The topic of conversation is now shifting generally to the intersection between religion and capital punishment, and specifically to the place that religious themes and activities occupy in our death penalty practices.[25]

It is a very common practice, especially in closing arguments, for prosecutors to make use of religious quotations or allusions in an effort to secure a death verdict from a jury.[26] The most popular line of attack in this vein is to draw quotations from Mosaic law, and, not surprisingly, the classic retributive mantra of 'an eye for an eye' has proven to be a mainstay in this effort.[27] Other prosecutors have gone beyond simply seeking theological support for a man-imposed sanction of death, and instead tried to explicitly cloak the desired death verdict with divine authority. For example, a prosecutor in a Mississippi capital case referred to himself as, "the servant of God to execute [H]is wrath on the wrongdoer[,]"[28] while another in Alabama referred to the jury as, "the tool of the Lord."[29] A third way in which prosecutors have used religious references to encourage a jury to return a sentence of death has been to offer comments on the religiosity of the victim and/or the defendant. As one might expect, prosecutorial comments regarding the religious character of victims have sought to place the victims on the right side of the higher power through such tactics as suggesting that a victim was "going up the ladder [to heaven,]"[30] speculating that the victims in a multiple homicide were praying when they were killed,[31] and claiming that the victims in another double murder case were, "good honest hardworking God fearing people."[32] The comments regarding the religiosity of defendants, on the other hand, have generally taken the form of either casting aspersions on the sincerity of the defendant's purported religious beliefs[33] or suggesting that a defendant would be highly encouraged to, "get his soul right"[34] or "repent"[35] as a result of being put under the threat of a pending execution.

Defense attorneys, like prosecutors, are also prone to invoke religious language and imagery in their comments to capital jurors. Of course, consistent with their function, defense counsel use religion in an attempt to avoid a sentence of death for their clients. These efforts generally take the form of stories from the Bible to illustrate that mercy is a basic value of Christian belief[36] or references to biblical passages that seem to prohibit capital punishment in an attempt to counter the 'eye for an eye' retributive argument from the prosecution.[37] Additionally, defense counsel frequently interject religion into the proceedings by putting on proof of the defendant's religious beliefs and actions as evidence in mitigation.[38] It is generally this evidence that prosecutors are attacking when they engage in the aforementioned casting of aspersions on the sincerity of the defendant's religiosity.

Beyond the efforts of prosecutors and defense attorneys, there are other ways in which religious themes are interjected into the trial court proceedings of death penalty cases. Two of these avenues are through the presentation of victim impact testimony and the efforts of individual jurors. Victim impact testimony is presented to capital juries as a means of impressing upon the jurors the uniqueness of the individual whose life has been taken by the defendant. One way of accomplishing this goal that is generally believed to be effective at building up empathy for the victim is to present evidence and testimony that the victim was a devout religious adherent. For example, in a Georgia capital case victim impact testimony was elicited which claimed that the murder victim had, "new found faith and spirituality" and was a "dedicated member of his church family ..."[39] Similarly, family members of the victims in a Louisiana triple murder prosecution, testified that religion was paramount in the victims' lives and that the victims were extremely dedicated to the Catholic Church.[40]

Perhaps inspired by the religious-laden speech of prosecutors, defense attorneys and victim impact witnesses, some jurors have taken it upon themselves to give their deliberations religious overtones. In the California case of People v. Mincey, a juror brought a Bible into the deliberation room after a lunch recess in order to, in that juror's words, show the other jurors that there were, "different views [about capital punishment] that come from the Bible."[41] A more partisan use of religion was employed by a member of the jury in a South Carolina capital case, when a juror circulated a pamphlet titled 'God, Law, and Capital Punishment', which expressed a pro-death penalty view and included references to Bible passages to support that view.[42] Consistent with these occurrences within the courtroom, it is not uncommon to find explicit interaction between religion and the death penalty in other death penalty practices.

Of course, as criminal law in the United States is predominately the creature of statutory codes, if a jurisdiction is to have the death penalty, that authority must come from the appropriate legislative body. When legislators are called upon to approve the death penalty for their constituencies, they, at times, attempt to cloak their decisions with divine authority. For example, when Texas adopted its death penalty statute in 1973 a debate erupted between legislators over the appropriateness of capital punishment from the Christian point-of-view. One opponent of the bill commented that state executions violated the Ten Commandments' prohibition on killing, only to be met with a response from the bill's three co-sponsors that consisted of citing Biblical passages which they believed supported the death penalty.[43]

At the end of the timeline that governs capital punishment, the public are frequently presented with a picture of religion and the death penalty residing side-by-side on death rows and in death chambers. Many reports out of death row tell of condemned prisoners spending their last hours on earth engaged in religious activities. For example, a press account of Karla Faye Tucker's 1998 execution in Texas, reported how Ms. Tucker read the Bible and prayed with her family and the prison warden while she awaited her lethal injection.[44] Thereafter, once inside the death chamber and facing their imminent demise, the last words uttered by many of the condemned are often steeped in the language of religion. Common refrains heard from defendants at this point include declarations of a belief in God, prayers for forgiveness and repentance, and claims that the prisoner will soon be in a better place.[45] From here, the entire effort is often capped off by the state officials responsible for the execution including religious comments in their final words on the matter: when, then Texas Governor, George W. Bush addressed the public after Ms. Tucker's execution, he spoke of leaving matters of the heart and soul to, "a higher authority", stated that he had sought, "guidance through prayer", and closed with the words, "May God bless Karla Faye Tucker and may God bless her victims and their families."[46] Later, in the summer of 2000, as Governor Bush was in the midst of a tough race for the U.S. Presidency, he presided over the highly publicized execution of Gary Graham and once again invoked the name of God in his remarks. After claiming that he was confident in Mr. Graham's guilt, an issue that was being debated widely in the days leading up to the execution, Mr. Bush, as he had done in the Tucker case, invoked God's blessing on the event by saying, "May God bless the victims, the families of the victims, and God bless Mr. Graham."[47]

The ultimate effect of the pervasive intertwining that exists between our death penalty practices and religion is that the latter legitimates the former, and thus serves to mask the evil that underlies our capital punishment system. The ability of religion to legitimate social institutions is a phenomenon well known to the social sciences. Religion accomplishes this task by bestowing upon these institutions a sacred and cosmic status. Through the process of religious legitimisation human activity is related positively to the ultimate, universal and sacred reality that underlies fervently held religious beliefs. The identification of human action with this divine cosmos means that those actions take on a rightness that is normally associated with the higher power itself. In this fashion, human government and punishment, for example, become sacramental phenomena and are seen as channels through which divine forces are made to impinge upon the lives of men. These human institutions are given a semblance of inevitability, firmness and durability that is normally reserved for what is sacred and divine, and thus, they pass into the realm of the inevitable.

The exact process just described was plainly on display when the prosecutor from Mississippi referred to himself as being an instrument of God's wrath, and when the Alabama prosecutor called upon the jury to see itself as God's "tool." This is also the case with individual jurors in capital cases and the co-sponsors of the Texan death penalty legislation who cite Biblical passages to support the sanction, and with (then) Governor Bush who in his post-execution remarks talks of deferring to a "higher power", praying for guidance, and calling for God's blessing to be passed upon the executed prisoners and their victims. In all these instances religion was invoked to take a man-created official exercise of violence and transform it into a function of a higher power whose rightness is largely beyond question. Although to a lesser degree, a defense counsel making a religious argument against capital punishment and a condemned prisoner praying and praising God just before his or her death, also serve to legitimate the death penalty. The defense counsel's arguments help locate the debate over the rightness of capital punishment on a plane that enables us to disown some of the responsibility that should accompany the deliberate killing of others. That is, the matter takes on the character of a theological debate as opposed to a moral dilemma. The religious activities of the condemned on the other hand, mask the evil of the event by encouraging us to see the conversion of the prisoner as the culmination of a divinely inspired effort to redeem one of our most wayward sinners as opposed to the premeditated killing of another.

2.   Conclusion

We have arrived at the point of seeing the death penalty as an act of evil that survives in America, in part, because our society takes some pains to avoid confronting the full consequence of that sanction. By hiding the evil that underlies the process of capital punishment, the participation of professionals, and religion, we manage to lessen the moral quandary that is presented by the death penalty, thus allowing the sanction to survive and prosper. But this survival is not without cost.

In crass economic terms it is well established that taking the average capital defendant from trial through to execution costs more money that taking the average capital defendant from trial through a lifetime sentence.[48] So, if we measure the profitableness of our criminal justice efforts in dollars and cents, the death penalty is a losing proposition. This economic cost however, is a minor debit on society's ledger when compared with the intangible costs that are incurred by our continued use of capital punishment.

A system that doles out state-sanctioned killings under the influence of incompetent counsel and racial bias cannot help but be corrupting. A system that subjects some innocent citizens to the possibility of an undeserved death and actually imposes the same on others cannot help but place the entire criminal justice process in contempt. More importantly, a system that intentionally pursues the death of others in order to satisfy some sense of vengeance or retribution inevitably cheapens our regard for life and erodes our self respect.

Notes

1. Floyd, 2001, 945; Radelet, 2000, 9; Radelet & Akers, 1996, 3.
2. van den Haag, 1985, 966.
3. Holmes, 1897, 469.
4. Greenberg, 1986, 1677.
5. Bright, 1994, 1835.
6. McClesky v. Kemp, 481 U.S. 279 (1987); Bassett, 2002, 31.
7. Radelet et al., 1992.
8. Gottlieb, 1989, 457.
9. Johnson, 1998, 50.
10. Campbell v. Wood, 18 F.3d 662, 683 (9th Cir. 1994).
11. Cabana, 1996, 158 & 161-63.
12. Marquart et al., 1994, 234-40.
13. Bessler, 1997, 149-50.
14. Johnson, 47.
15. Bright, 1995, 1212-16; Bright & Keenan, 1995, 769-76.
16. Raedker-Jordan, 1996, 537-44.
17. Martin, 1997, 125-28.

18. Haney, 1997, 1484.
19. Haney, 1481.
20. Howarth, 1994, 1410-11.
21. Haney, 1456-69.
22. Mello, 1997, 200-04.
23. Michalos, 1997, 126-27; Council on Ethical & Judicial Affairs, 1993, 365.
24. Ford v. Wainwright, 477 U.S. 408, 409-10 (1986).
25. Although the following paragraphs focus exclusively on the contemporary intersection between religion and the death penalty, this is not meant to suggest that this is a relatively new phenomenon. The intertwining of religion and state-sanctioned executions is a practice with a very long pedigree. Banner, 2002, 16-22 & 32-36; Douglas, 2000, 137.
26. Simson & Garvey, 2001, 1110; Blume & Johnson, 2000, 64.
27. Ibid ; Ibid, 64-65.
28. Berry v. State, 703 So. 2d 269, 281 (Miss. 1997).
29. McNair v. State, 653 So. 2d 320, 339 (Ala. Crim. App. 1992).
30. Cape v. Francis, 71 F.2d 1287, 1301 (11th Cir. 1984).
31. State v. Ramsey, 864 S.W.2d 320, 332 (Mo. 1993).
32. Lucas v. Evatt, 416 S.E.2d 646, 648 (S.C. 1992).
33. Blume & Johnson, 68-69.
34. People v. Sandoval, 841 P.2d 862, 883 (Cal. 1982).
35. People v. Wrest, 839 P.2d 1020, 1028 (Cal. 1992).
36. Blume & Johnson, 71-72.
37. Simson & Garvey, 1110; Blume & Johnson, 72-73.
38. People v. Payton, 839 P.2d 1035, 1040 (Cal.1992).
39. Turner v. State, 486 S.E.2d 839, 842 (Ga. 1997).
40. State v. Koon, 704 So. 2d 756, 773-74 (La. 1997).
41. 827 P.2d 388, 424 (Cal. 1992).
42. State v. Kelly, 502 S.E.2d 99, 103 n. 3 (S.C. 1998).
43. Holberg v. State, 38 S.W.3d 137, 139 (Tex. Crim. App. 2000).
44. Ward & Rodriguez, 1998, A1.s
45. Texas Department of Corrections, 2002, www.
46. Herman, 1998, A1.
47. Mills & Pearson, 2000, 1.
48. Drehle, 1995, 358.

References

Banner, S. (2002), *The Death Penalty: An American History*. Cambridge: Harvard University Press.

Bassett, T. (2002), 'Risking Cruelty: McCleskey v. Kemp, Retributivism, and Ungrounded Moral Judgment'. *Syracuse Law Review*. 52: 1-49.

Berger, P.L. (1969), *The Social Reality of Religion*. London: Faber.

Berry v. State, 703 So. 2d 269 (Miss. 1997).

Bessler, J.D. (1997), *Death in the Dark: Midnight Executions in America*. Boston: Northeastern University Press.

Blume, J.H. and S.L. Johnson (2000), 'Don't Take His Eye, Don't Take His Tooth, and Don't Cast the First Stone: Limiting Religious Arguments in Capital Cases'. *William and Mary Bill of Rights Journal*, 9: 61-104.

Bright, S.B. (1995), 'The Death Penalty as the Answer to Crime: Costly, Counterproductive, and Corrupting'. *Santa Clara Law Review*. 35: 1211-36.

Bright, S.B. and P.J. Keenan (1995), 'Judges and the Politics of Death: Deciding Between the Bill of Rights and the Next Election in Capital Cases'. *Boston University Law Review*. 75: 759-835.

Bright, S.B. (1994), 'Counsel for the Poor: The Death Sentence Not for the Worst Crime But for the Worst Lawyer'. *Yale Law Journal*. 103: 1835-83.

Cabana, D.A. (1996), *Death at Midnight: The Confession of an Executioner*. Boston: Northeastern University Press.

Campbell v. Wood, 18 F.3d 662 (9th Cir. 1994).

Cape v. Francis, 71 F.2d 1287 (11th Cir. 1984).

Council on Ethical & Judicial Affairs, AMA (21 July, 1993), 'Physician Participation in Capital Punishment'. *Journal of American Medical Association*. 365-68.

Douglas, D.M. (2000), 'God and the Executioner: The Influence of Western Religion on the Death Penalty'. *William and Mary Bill of Rights Journal*. 9: 137-70.

Floyd, T.W. (2001), ' "'What's Going On?'": Christian Ethics and the

Modern American Death Penalty'. *Texas Tech Law Review*. 32: 931-53.
Ford v. Wainwright, 477 U.S. 408 (1986).

Gottlieb, D.J. (1989), 'The Death Penalty in the Legislature: Some
Thoughts About Money, Myth, and Morality'. *University of Kansas Law
Review*. 37: 443-70.

Greenberg, J. (1986), 'Against the American System of Capital
Punishment'. *Harvard Law Review*. 99: 1670-80.

Haney, C. (1997), 'Violence and the Capital Jury: Mechanisms of Moral
Disengagement and the Impulse to Condemn to Death'. *Stanford Law
Review*. 49: 1447-86.

Herman, K. (Feb. 4, 1998), 'Bush Decision Unlikely to Have Political
Fallout'. *Austin American-Statesman*. A1.

Holberg v. State, 38 S.W.3d 137 (Tex. Crim. App. 2000).

Holmes, O.W. (1897), 'The Path of the Law'. 10 *Harvard Law Review*.
10: 457-78.
Howarth, J.W. (1994), 'Deciding to Kill: Revealing the Gender in the
Task Handed to Capital Jurors'. *Wisconsin Law Review*, 1345-1424.

Johnson, R. (2d ed. 1998), *Death Work: A Study of the Modern Execution
Process*. Pacific Grove, California: Brooks/Cole.

Lucas v. Evatt, 416 S.E.2d 646 (S.C. 1992).

Marquart, J.W., S. Ekland-Olson and J.R. Sorenson (1994), *The Rope, The
Chair, and The Needle: Capital Punishment in Texas, 1923-1990*. Austin:
University of Texas Press.

Martin, E.F. (1997), 'Towards an Evolving Debate on the Decency of
Capital Punishment'. *George Washington Law Review*. 66: 84-134.

McClesky v. Kemp, 481 U.S. 279 (1987).

McNair v. State, 653 So. 2d 320 (Ala. Crim. App. 1992).

Mello, M.A. (1997), *Dead Wrong: A Death Row Lawyer Speaks Out
Against Capital Punishment*. Madison: University of Wisconsin Press.

Michalos, C. (1997), 'Medical Ethics and the Execution Process in the United States of America'. *Medicine and Law.* 16: 125-163.

Mills, S. and R. Pearson (June 23, 2000), 'Texas Executes Graham'. *Chicago Tribune.* 1.

People v. Mincey, 827 P.2d 388 (Cal. 1992).

People v. Payton, 839 P.2d 1035 (Cal.1992).

People v. Sandoval, 841 P.2d 862 (Cal. 1982).

People v. Wrest, 839 P.2d 1020 (Cal. 1992).

Raedker-Jordan, S. (1996), 'A Pro-Death, Self-Fulfilling Constitutional Construct: The Supreme Court's Evolving Standard of Decency for the Death Penalty'. *Hastings Constitutional Law Quarterly.* 23: 455-556.

Radelet, M.L. (2000), 'The Role of Organized Religions in Changing Death Penalty Debates'. *William and Mary Bill of Rights Journal.* 9: 201-14.

Radelet, M.L., H.A Bedau and C.E. Putnam (1992), *In Spite of Innocence: Erroneous Convictions in Capital Cases.* Boston: Northeastern University Press.

Radelet, M.L. and R.L Akers (1996), 'Deterrence and the Death Penalty: The Views of the Experts'. *Journal of Criminal Law and Criminology.* 87: 1-16.

Simson, G.J. and S.P. Garvey (2001), 'Knockin' on Heaven's Door: Rethinking the Role of Religion in Death Penalty Cases'. *Cornell Law Review*, 86: 1090-1130.

State v. Kelly, 502 S.E.2d 99 (S.C. 1998).

State v. Koon, 704 So. 2d 756 (La. 1997).
State v. Ramsey, 864 S.W.2d 320 (Mo. 1993).

Texas Department of Corrections, (1 March, 2002), 'Executed Offenders'. http://www.tdcj.state.tx.us/stat/executedoffenders.htm.

Turner v. State, 486 S.E.2d 839 (Ga. 1997).

van den Haag, E. (1985), 'The Death Penalty Once More'. *University of California at Davis Law Review*. 18: 957-72.

Drehle, D.V. (1995), *Among the Lowest of the Dead: The Culture of Death Row*. New York: Times Books.

Ward, M. and R. Rodriquez (1998), 'Texas Executes Tucker', *Austin American-Statesman*, A1. 4 Feb.

Interrogating the Penal Gaze: Is the Ethical Prison a Possibility?

Diana Medlicott

In so-called advanced societies, the prison has emerged historically as the principle form of punishment. Most of us know surprisingly little about prisons, because until recently they were closed off from the rest of society. More recently however, the prison has become a cultural artefact as well as a form of punishment. It is the subject of books, films, plays and other forms of mass entertainment. Partly because of this, and partly because the prison has become somewhat more accessible to the media and the general public, we think that we know much more about prison life. We know that the prison is a world where the inmates are confined against their will, and governed systematically so that they have to surrender autonomy and conform to the rules in a pared-down existence.

At the same time, we know that prisons are violent and frightening places, and that inmates generally emerge hardened and possibly brutalised by the experience of incarceration. So we need to be able to justify putting fellow citizens into such a world. If prison can be made to fit with a sustainable theory of justification, then it can be claimed as a legitimate part of our moral and political order.

1.   Prison and The Crisis of Legitimacy

The prison as the principle form of punishment in modern societies is suffering a crisis of legitimacy on two levels. The first is at the conceptual level of justification and the second is concerned with the empirical operation of the prison, including its effects. These two levels are linked, in that we cannot conceptually approve the principle of justification if the empirical evidence falsifies the principle. So, for instance, we cannot justify the prison on the grounds that it is rehabilitative if, in practice, it manifestly and consistently fails to rehabilitate.

Whether we adopt a utilitarian or retributive perspective, it is difficult to justify this particular manner of doing intentional harm to fellow citizens. As deterrence, prison patently does not work on either an individual or a general level, as the re-offending rates indicate. However, prison does not only fail to reform on a significant level: the overwhelming evidence is that it also succeeds in actually making people worse. The retributive argument is also hard to sustain, because it is backward looking and returns harm for harm. Retributivists might argue that retribution deters, but there is not a shred of evidence that this is the case. It is also hard to agree on what amount of punishment is an appropriate and just dessert for any given crime and for any given offender. Retributive punishment can look suspiciously like raw vengeance. Given these fundamental ambiguities, it is hard to locate retribution in an ethical framework. The lack of consensus on what is appropriate can be illustrated by two particular cases. In the first case, a seventy-eight year old man in the UK has recently been sentenced to a week in prison for not paying his community charge. In sunny California, a man has received a sentence of twenty-five years to life for stealing a tyre. It was his third 'strike'. His previous two 'strikes' were in the 1970s and 1980s.

One way in which we could sustain a justification for the prison as punishment would be if we could show that the prison itself was an ethical entity in the way in which it operated. As an ethical universe in miniature, such an institution would contain all the grounds necessary for producing good rather than harmful effects. Is an ethical prison possible? To answer this question, I am going to narrow my discussion to consider the realm of the visual. Like other institutions set up to deal with specialised populations, the prison awards a special sort of attention to its inmates: we can describe this attention as an attentive gaze. It looks at its clientele in a particular way and the look expresses a certain kind of attention.

The modern prison emerged in a new post Enlightenment scientific age, when knowledge of all kinds was developing into a range of practices used to manage human beings who presented particular problems. There was a growth in types of authoritative gaze - the look informed with knowledge that gazed upon a particular group of persons and declared authoritatively what was wrong with them and what should be done to them.[1] The new medical gaze, for instance, soon came to possess a kind of sovereign power and it extended that power from scrutiny and treatment of physical illness to that of mental illness.[2] Visual experience and the informed look were crucial in diagnosis and management: the power to look, with special knowledge, became the power that could bring truth to light. The penal gaze has remorselessly extended its remit and the last 200 years have seen an ever-increasing administrative apparatus, bureaucratic expansion and professionalization.[3]

2.   The Visual Order and the Seeing Eye of Panopticon
Vision is a primordial capacity. Our language is saturated with visual metaphors. We cannot reflect on the past, have insight in the present or dream of the future except by recourse to the concept of the visual. Vision is additionally reflexive. How we see the Other is productive of how we

treat the Other, and in turn this produces particular responses to us by the Other.

Up until the end of the 18th century, prisons were not places where a specific ideological gaze looked intently at individuals. They had tended to be chaotic places where the inmates mingled relatively freely with each other. Jeremy Bentham's panoptic vision, at the end of the 18th century, of a specially designed institution with separate cells, is often taken both as a departure from this trend and a reflection of the modern prison. In his 1791 treatise on a model prison, Bentham envisaged a circular arrangement of cells: in the centre was a tower with a jailor in it. The jailor himself could see into all the cells, but shutters prevented the prisoners from returning his gaze and seeing him. This was a sinister embodiment of the unreciprocal visual dialectic.[4] The gaze itself was invisible, but it saw all that there was to see.

What does the penal gaze say to those it looks upon? It says, quite clearly, that you are the objects of my gaze, but you are no longer the subject who can return look for look: you cannot look back at me. In one stroke, the humanity of the visual subject is destroyed. It is no coincidence that, in Orwell's *1984*, one of the most painfully experienced negations of humanity is the Seeing Eye in the corner of the living room.

The new 19th century prisons had cells of a uniform size. There were rules of silence, solitary confinement, religious instruction and labour discipline. The prison was in Bentham's vision, a mill for grinding rogues honest. Sometimes prisoners had to wear masks or headgear, which prevented them from looking at one another. They would be put into individual boxed cages with small slits to look out of and made to listen to lectures on sobriety and virtue. They could only face ahead: they could not look at anyone or anything but the lecturer. Punishment became thoroughly calculated, controlled, measured and bureaucratised. It became calibrated, rather like Bentham's whipping machine. Bentham's whipping machine may have focused on the body, but what it shared with the panoptic prison was its intentional reduction of the human subject to a mere object or thing, to be practiced upon and forced to comply. The panoptic prison did this efficiently by envisioning prisoners as objects, controlling their visual capacities, and finally by encouraging prisoners to construe themselves in degraded ways.

This control of the visual realm was only one aspect of the rational management of populations in the modern age. It was new knowledge, and it sought objects on which to practice. The strategic planning and rational administration of prisons point to a peculiar combination in the modern age of knowledge and power. This was a technology of control, with its own internal logic. Cultural traits and the sensibilities of any given society at a particular time can ameliorate that technology of control. It may, for instance, be ameliorated more generously at times of economic strength and expansion, but however attenuated the overt control, there is an underlying force that demands compliance, built on specialist knowledge and practices.

For the most part, in so-called advanced societies, the prison operates an economy of power: it does not need to torture, whip or bludgeon. It can achieve its effects with far milder expression. Bodies are placed in cells so that they occupy *that* slot and no other and timetables indicate the slot of time they are to occupy. The bodies are fed, exercised, and trained inasmuch as resources allow. Bodies are released when their time is served. If bodies escape the sentence through self-inflicted death or leaping over the walls, it is a serious discipline matter. Someone is at fault, because they failed to invigilate intensely enough: through a failure in watching and seeing, they did not manage to keep the body living and breathing, and in its allotted space and time.[5]

Foucault reminds us that the birth of the modern prison occurred alongside the major technology of the telescope, the lens and the light beam: "using techniques of subjection and methods of exploitation, an obscure art of light and the visible was secretly preparing a new knowledge of man".[6] The prison, with its emphasis on surveillance, was the forerunner of closed circuit television, speed cameras and other Orwellian ways of reducing human subjects to the object of systematic scrutiny.

3.   The Object of the Gaze
Who is the object of the penal gaze?

The striking characteristic of the post-Enlightenment discourses concerned with managing special populations is that the authoritative gaze does not see a given and objective reality, which would be seen by, for instance, the untrained layperson or the unschooled child. The 'reality' seen by a special gaze can only be seen because the gaze is intentional and armed with special knowledge. Any one of these gazes both constructs and 'sees' an epistemic field. This field is constructed linguistically, just as importantly as through vision.[7] And so the penal gaze over the next centuries would problematise whole populations, casting them as appropriate objects for isolation from society, placing them so that they could be invigilated in ways that did not permit a reciprocal scrutiny.

What do we find when we look at the objects of the penal gaze in terms of whole populations? We find the poor, the unemployed, the stateless, the marginalized, the refugee, the socially excluded, and the economic migrant all forming prison populations worldwide. Inmate populations all over the world reflect the systemic discrimination of the particular society with regard to indigenous people and ethnic minorities. Thus, whilst aboriginal people in Canada amount to three percent of the general population, they form seventeen percent of the federal inmate population.[8] In the USA, about a third of young African American males are under one or other form of criminal justice sanction on any particular day, and about one in eight black males is incarcerated.[9] In Western Australia, indigenous youth form under four percent of the youth population, yet at any one time between fifty and sixty percent of children and young people in custody in this state will be aboriginal.[10]

These patterned occurrences of racial and ethnic disproportionality in prison populations all over the world are living examples of Foucault's thesis about the constitutive capacity of power and knowledge. If we mistakenly construe power as a negative force that excludes, represses, masks and conceals, we miss its true identity. Power is constitutive: it creates domains of objects. The panoply of power and discipline, the range of surveillance techniques, and the rationalising practices are all part of a strategy of power relations.[11]

As well as constituting populations and domains of objects, power also creates individuals. Power individualises, and knowledge of the individual is gained and practiced to produce real effects.[12] So, if we move up closer to the populations in prison, what are the personal characteristics of these individual objects of the penal gaze? The most defining characteristics of the majority of people in prison belong to the discourse of need. Let us leave aside here those few powerful, autonomous individuals who apparently choose a self and wilfully live it in defiant and conscious rebellion against society's norms. We might argue about who falls into this category, but what is unarguable is that most people in prison lack full autonomy; they are weak, damaged and marginalized, socially, economically, and/or politically.

Let us consider the example of women in prison in the UK. Few of them have ever had paid employment; most have at least one of the following indicators of damage - a history of sexual and/or physical abuse, substance abuse or addiction, mental disorder, a childhood in care, a lack of basic education, a history of self-harm. But over seventy percent have never been in prison before, so it appears that the prison is usefully mopping up these pitiably needy women and keeping them out of our sight for a measure of time.[13] Of course, the penal gaze does not construe them as needy. It construes them as blame-worthy and deserving of punishment and exclusion.

This perception, that the objects of the penal gaze are less human than the law-abiding majority, is the result of historical changes in representation. The birth of the modern prison gave us an image of the criminal and the prisoner: through a collective acquiescence in the face of powerful discourses, we arrived at an intentional visualisation of these objects. In prison, inmates are often referred to as bodies; officers talk about 'feeding' them. Quite casually and not necessarily with much overt hostility, officers routinely objectify prisoners in derogatory language. This is a taken-for-granted mode of seeing, and society sustains it to some extent. It is assumed that we do not want to look at these worthless objects, and thanks to a collective human will operating over several centuries, they have been removed from our sight. The vast river of need in prisoners, the social and economic deficits, the psychological damage, the pain-filled biographies and the lack of stability in their lives are also hidden from our sight. We do not have to think about prisoners except as objects of the penal gaze.

How does the individual self construe itself once it has been construed and envisioned as an object? The answer is that it begins to see itself, quite quickly, in the blinding reflective light of the authoritative gaze, as a degraded thing. It is true that there are people who experience prison, and somehow manage to transcend its effects. By extraordinary acts, they turn their lives around and manage to re-construct themselves as ethical subjects. But, for most, the prison experience is productive of profound shame. Even when prisoners are aware of the strategies designed to objectify and humiliate them, they find it hard to resist the powerful shaming effects.[14]

Let us now make a little digression into the visual domain of the prison. It is a Tuesday afternoon in early January. I am sitting in a cell on a cardboard chair, beside the bed of a young man of eighteen called Thomas. Thomas has refused to leave his cell for over three months, either for education, exercise or even to collect his meals from the serving hatch at the far end of the wing. At mealtimes, the other inmates are unlocked and go to collect their meal. Every meal, the officers unlock his cell, and he remains inside. He has not had a meal for three months, or a shower. The officers will not deliver the meal to his cell, a distance of about twenty feet from the serving hatch, because the rules clearly state that inmates must collect their own food and take it back to their cells. The only time Thomas has left his cell is when he was forcibly removed because of a fire drill. He was then charged with disobeying an order and put in the segregation unit for a few days before being returned to his cell. His cell contains a lavatory and a wash hand basin. Thomas has sufficient money to continue buying his weekly canteen allowance via a standard form. Every week, items up to about £4 in value are delivered to his cell, and thus he is surviving on biscuits and packet soups that he mixes up with hot water from his washbasin.

Thomas's arm and leg muscles are visibly wasted, he is pale and non-communicative. He intends to serve the remaining five months in this fashion. He is keeping his cell clean and himself too. He shaves most days and does not smell too bad. Thinking out loud, I tell him that he reminds me of a soldier, hiding out in the woods after a war, living a pared down life that only thinks of survival. A curious expression flits across his face, perhaps of pride? He smiles faintly, looks at me directly (which is rare) and does not reply, but a flicker of some kind of understanding seems to pass between us.

On this particular afternoon, Thomas is quite talkative. As he talks, lying flat on his bed with an arm over his eyes, my eyes roam around the cell. He is choosing not to see as he talks, and I am looking to see what he sees when he does choose to look around him. I start my scrutiny of the cell at the top right-hand corner and move my gaze leftward, over the bars on the high dirty window, through which I can see something grey, indistinct and dismal that I can almost believe is the sky. Almost immediately my eyes reach the left hand corner, and as they slip down the bleak wall, I see various spots and stains that look like vomit, shit and blood. At the bottom of the wall is a washbasin, and my eyes widen with relief because here at last is some colour. On the basin stands a small box of powdered soup packets, each of which can be mixed up in a cup with hot water from the tap. The box of soup packets is a comforting red colour, and the red cardboard has a dull little gleam in the gloom of the cell. From the basin, my eyes roam leftward and when I turn my head, quite quickly my vision hits the third corner. Behind me is the great clanging door to the cell and to the right behind me are the lavatory and the last corner of the cell. That brings us right round the cell and back to my vantage point beside the bed. Restlessly, as Thomas speaks in a monotonous, slow voice, my eyes begin again their perambulation around the cell. Always, the red cardboard box of powdered soup is a relief for my eyes. Even so, after an hour, I become aware of a visual craving. I long to look at colour, light, and interesting objects. I want to stretch my eyes - look at a vista that is longer than four or five feet. How, I wonder, would I last in a cell with this restriction to the primordial sense of seeing?

Driving home along the motorway later that day, across great tracts of middle England countryside, my eyes roam hungrily across the ploughed land, the woodland, and the extraordinary winter sky. The freedom to stare, now at something small and compact like a Hereford cow, now at something in the distance like a wooded copse on the curve of a hill, seems intoxicating in its variety. I think of Thomas in his small space, with its degraded opportunities for seeing. I wonder if he finds any visual relief in the red box of powdered soups, or if he has fashioned for himself other visual compensations.

Thinking about Thomas, I come to see him as an object of the penal gaze who is struggling not to capitulate. He does not want to become an object. He has very few avenues open to him in which to express his autonomy and his status as a human subject. He could fight and become really violent and embark upon the revolving door of many young prisoners as they get shuffled from segregation unit to segregation unit, in prisons up and down the country. He could spend hours sawing at his wrists and arms, pushing paper clips into veins. He could attempt hanging and fasting, as other prisoners do. But Thomas has not chosen these ways. He does not want to cause trouble: he just wants to resist being objectified. He has chosen to exercise control over the issue of why and when he comes out of his cell. He can decide very little for himself in prison, but this he will decide. By remaining wilfully in his cell, he is exercising autonomy and control over his life by one of the few means left to him.

In my research in prisons, I have come across innumerable examples of prisoners who struggle to remain autonomous subjects. Once, with a blaze of passion, a man convicted of several horrific rapes, told me that he, and he alone, can decide when his heart stops beating. From time to time, he attempted suicide, not because he wanted to die, but because he wanted to remind himself of his capacity to choose a fate and remain a deciding subject.

The destruction of autonomy, which is accomplished so economically in most modern prisons, although there are some golden exceptions, is made possible by the original gaze, which looked upon its objects and constituted them as less than fully human.[15] This gaze is enabled to practice in prisons by forms of architecture, rules and codes of conduct. Here is one small example: as I move up and down the wings, I can look into any cell I want. All I need to do is open the flap on the outside of the heavy cell door. As I peer through, the prisoner may well be using the lavatory in his cell. He cannot choose not to be watched: there is no flap on his side of the door, which he can open or close at will. He will be watched or not watched, but he may not ever choose. This is because he has been constituted as the object of a gaze, a gaze that he may not return because he has lost his right to reciprocate this most natural of human activities. Visual innocence and neutrality have been destroyed: with the gaze comes a judgement about a field of objects. It does not wait to judge, on the basis of experience. It judges because its function is to judge.

4.   Conclusion

In this chapter, I have isolated some aspects of historical process in order to interrogate the notion of the ethical prison. I have done this by a narrow focus upon vision and the capacity of the penal gaze. Culturally we tend to think of vision and the gaze as 'natural' capacities, grounded in physiology, forgetting the intentionalist aspects which, when enacted in historical change, seem to take on the nature of a collective will.[16] The nature of the look, as applied to problem populations, determines how truth is recognised, errors are avoided, judgements are made and knowledge is built up. So vision, as the look which envisions the Other and decides how to act in relation to the Other, is an epistemic quality.

In its view of what prisoners are, the penal gaze, as exemplified by the prison, is essentially flawed. This flaw is epistemic, because the way in which the penal gaze construes the prisoner results in the practice of a knowledgeable discourse which construes prisoners as objects of a particular sort. This construal produces real effects in terms of how the prisoner is housed and treated and it leads on to the prisoner construing him or herself in particular degrading ways.

Could we correct this epistemic flaw in the penal gaze? Could we then, as a result, re-construct the prison empirically, and in so doing restore the security of a justification that would resolve the crisis of legitimacy over the prison as the principle form of punishment? Is the ethical prison a possibility? What might an ethical prison look like? At its very least, I suggest that it would be a community where the self is allowed to respect and care for itself, exercise autonomy, respect others and work toward a mastery of those capacities required to function lawfully in civil society.

The first necessary change involves the very nature of the penal gaze. It must cease to construe prisoners as objects and as the inevitable repositories for moral vices. The expectation that individuals will behave badly on any given occasion and in any given context, must be abandoned, and a different set of expectations must define policy. Prisoners must be construed as human subjects imbued with sets of different possibilities. The offences for which they have been apprehended only represent one kind of possibility, but do not drive out the others. When individuals behave well, the penal gaze has trouble in recognising virtue, in the same way that the medical gaze, intent upon finding evidence of mental illness, finds it hard to recognise mental health and construes even 'normal' behaviour as pathological.[17] So the penal gaze constructs a non-virtuous universe, and looks upon its inhabitants as unworthy objects in that universe.

In an ethical universe, the penal gaze would abandon its addiction to punishment. It would cease to be 'penal': it would become an expectant look that sought reciprocity. This expectant gaze would construct a institutional universe where virtues would play a central role. We could not call this place prison: let us call it Possibility. In Possibility, the expectant gaze would be intent upon constructing the moral subject, through choice and the exercise of autonomy. Offenders in the Possibility community would share responsibility, with staff, for ordering life inside the closed community, for decision-making, for setting rules, for organising and distributing resources and for penalising those who break the rules. The rules would be justified insofar as the conduct they endorse would be virtuous and beneficial for the community members. Inhabitants would be offered the services they need, in terms of confronting their offending behaviour, their motivation for harming others, the abuse and violence done to them in their lives hitherto, as well as mental health services, help with addiction and dependence, education, training and employment skills. They would be required to give up behaviour that compromised their autonomy in involuntary ways, such as drugs, violence, bullying and alcohol. If, over a period of time, they chose systematically to eschew the exercise of autonomy in positive ways, they would be re-located in an institution with pared down facilities, and serve a conventional sentence. This would be the possibility that they themselves had chosen. Because the desire and capacities for personal change ebb and flow at different times for different people, there should however, be regular opportunities for offenders to try and re-try life in the ethical community.

In this way, the inhabitants of this possible community would be autonomous agents. Upon release, they would not construe themselves as degraded objects, so they would be less likely to treat others as objects to be victimised.

It is over ten years since the Woolf Report in the UK pointed out that prisoners need to be treated with humanity and justice: treating them brutally only produces further brutal behaviour.[18] Even in former totalitarian countries, leaders are recognising, often from personal experience of imprisonment, that societies are strengthened and social bonds enriched when prisons are run virtuously. So the unthinkable is happening, and societies with a harsh record are starting to look honestly at that record.[19] All over the world, there are exciting initiatives happening: restorative justice initiatives are recognising the autonomy of offenders and victims alike, and giving each party an opportunity to participate as autonomous subjects in healing solutions. But in some societies like the UK, the penal gaze is simultaneously clinging on to its old ways of seeing, its degraded vision of prisoners as non-agents. In the UK, we are imprisoning more people than ever before. We imprison our citizens at a higher rate than countries such as Saudi Arabia or Turkey, whilst pouring scorn on their record of human rights abuses.

This chapter has focused on one aspect only of modern

imprisonment to argue that at the primordial level of the visual order, the prison is ethically compromised. The removal or curtailment of freedom is not of itself ethically compromising: it is justifiable in this domain, because it follows as a consequence of wrongdoing. Offenders may be said to 'choose' prison, in a sense, when they commit crimes, but these apparent choices are often constrained and shaped by personal biography, abusive childhoods, poverty, exclusion and psychological damage. So we must provide escape routes which will make up for the terrible deficits suffered and enable offenders to re-join society as fully participating citizens. If we offer these escape routes with positive expectation and full economic resources, we will be offering offenders the chance to practice freedom.

What cannot be ethically justified is the penal gaze and the way in which it constructs prisoners in its own image, whilst at the same time removing their capacity to practice freedom. In looking afresh at panopticism and Foucault's disciplinary thesis, I have argued that it is not the practices of power that make the ethical prison a contradiction in terms, but the visual impairment that epistemologically precedes and structures those practices of power. We must find another vision to inform our gaze when we look upon those who break our laws: we must keep a space for them to retain or acquire autonomy and we must make that space a virtuous one, in which the conditions of possibility exist for real personal change and subsequent social, political and economic inclusion.

Notes

1. See Foucault, 1979, for an account of the development of the prison as an actualisation of power and knowledge.
2. See Foucault 1965, for an account of this process.
3. See Garland, 1990, 177-192, for an account of the rationalization of punishment.
4. See Miller, 1975, 3-36 for a full account of Panopticon as the sinister embodiment of reason in surveillance.
5. See Foucault, 1979, 135-169, for an account of how bodies are made docile.
6. Ibid., 171.
7. For a development of argument, see Foucault, 1973.
8. Oades, 2001, 4-5.
9. Teague, 2001, 38-40.
10. Blagg, 2001, 15-16.
11. Foucault, 1979, 194.
12. Ibid.
13. Kenney-Herbert, 1999, 54-66.

14. See for example Medlicott, 2001, 107, where Marty and Bud discuss some of the 'ordinary' indignities of prison life.
15. See Shine 2000, for a multi-faceted account of Grendon Underwood, a therapeutic prison community where a respect for autonomy clearly informs the seeing eye of staff and prisoners.
16. See Jay, 1993, 381-434, for a rich exploration of this and other themes relating to visual culture and the history of ideas.
17. See Rosenhan, 1973, for a telling piece of research in this area.
18. Home Office, 1991.
19. Coyle, 2001, 6-7.

References

Blagg, H. (2001), 'Restorative Visions in Aboriginal Australia', *Criminal Justice Matters.* no. 44, pp. 15-17, CCJS.

Coyle, A. (2001), 'Justice Should Not End at the The Prison Gate', *Criminal Justice Matters.* no. 44, pp. 6-7, CCJS.

Foucault, M. (1965), *Madness and Civilisation.* Viking: New York.

Foucault, M. (1973), *The Birth of the Clinic: An Archaeology of Medical Perspectives.* Heinemann: London.

Foucault, M. (1979), *Discipline and Punish.* Penguin: Harmondsworth.

Garland, D. (1990), *Punishment and Modern Society.* Oxford University Press: Oxford.

Home Office (1991), *Prison Disturbances 1990 – The Woolf Report.* London: HMSO.

Kenney-Herbert, J. (1999), 'The Health Care of Women Prisoners in England and Wales: A Literature Review'. *Howard Journal of Criminal Justice,* 38:1, 54-66.

Jay, M. (1994), *Downcast Eyes: The Denigration of Vision in Twentieth Century French Thought.* London: UCLA Press

Oades, J. (2001), 'Global Trends in Corrections'. *Criminal Justice Matters.* No. 44, 4-5, CCJS.

Miller, J-A., (1975), 'Jeremy Bentham's Panoptic Device'. *Ornicar.* May, 3-36.

Rosenhan, D. (1973), 'On Being Sane in Unsane Places'. *Science,* 179.

Shine, J. (2000), *A Compilation of Grendon Research.* Aylesbury: HM Prison Grendon.

Teague, M. (2001), 'George W. Bush and the 'Texas Solution''. *Criminal Justice Matters.* No. 44, 38-40, CCJS.

The Contraction of the Heart: Anxiety, Radical Evil and Proximity in Patricia Highsmith's Ripley Novels

Fiona Peters

"Tom detested murder unless it was absolutely necessary."[1]

Patricia Highsmith was an American born writer who lived most of her life in Europe, dying in Switzerland in 1995. She is perhaps best known for the film adaptations of her novels, such as Hitchcock's *Strangers on a Train* (1951), and the recent *The Talented Mr. Ripley* (2000). Usually categorised as working within the crime fiction genre, Highsmith's work has confounded those readers and critics who prefer the crime novel to present clear-cut choices; reviews of her work over the fifty years of her writing career have constantly returned to the problem of whether she should be called a crime writer or a 'serious novelist'. Highsmith herself vacillated between caring and not caring about her categorisation, but, citing Dostoevsky as her favourite author, always argued that it is possible to use crime to investigate issues of ethics and morality: "since she thinks everyone has at one time imagined himself committing a crime, if not actually doing so, crime could be 'very good for illustrating moral points'."[2] Perhaps partly as a result of being labelled a crime fiction writer, Highsmith has been far less researched than might have been expected from so prodigious and interesting a writer: the only full length study so far, by Russell Harrison, is a reading her work through the perspective of Sartrian existentialism.

Highsmith's texts, in a way unique among writers working within the crime fiction genre, confront and expose the ambiguity at the heart of notions such as evil, ethics and human responsibility. She specialises in the portrayal of evil within her protagonists. For Highsmith, evil exists, and exists inside us all, irrespective of whether we recognise it within ourselves or not. She posits evil as an ever-present possibility and her work examines situations in which ordinary people find themselves face to face with this possibility. She argues: "I'm interested in the possibility of evil, of evil doings, in everybody, and the degree of it."[3]

In her novels Highsmith shows little or no interest in the so-called traditional crime genre format, where the hero is an agent representing 'good' against an evil or transgressive force. She is also less interested in the act of violence or murder in itself, than in the impulses, both internal and external, that lead to making evil choices. Most of her 'heroes' suffer from excessive guilt, usually leading to their downfall, whether or not their evil or wicked desires are actually acted upon. Highsmith claimed that her greatest interest in writing lay in her examination of guilt, summed up when she said: "What I am most interested in is the effect of guilt on my heroes, in good and evil existing in the same person."[4] However, throughout her work she recognises and takes into account the fact that the evil act never exists within a vacuum. It has consequences both for the perpetrator, the victim, and the broader community.

While Highsmith is primarily interested in the crippling nature of guilt and anxiety, Tom Ripley, arguably her most developed and best known 'hero', is a peculiarity within her work, a man who can live, happily, without these afflictions. The contrast between Highsmith's suffering 'heroes' and Tom Ripley's seeming lack of empathy towards others, which allows him to kill if the need arises, places Highsmith's writing in the arena of morality and ethical responsibility. Through her explorations of the aporetic nature of morality she shatters easy assumptions of good or bad, evil or moral codes of behaviour, negating the necessity for conventional, 'moral' heroes by refusing to make her work reflect an accepted moral standpoint.

The first Tom Ripley novel, *The Talented Mr Ripley* was published in 1955, and several of her other most powerful books written in the 1950s, encapsulate many of the issues and preoccupations of that time. While Tom Ripley follows the Jamesian tradition of leaving the United States for the seemingly freer European world, most of her other books from this period are set in America and scathingly criticise the conformity that was fed by the explosion of post War consumerism and the anxieties of the Cold war period.

An examination of the ways in which Highsmith challenges assumptions concerning ethical and moral behaviours leads into uncomfortable areas such as the possibility of radical evil as a foundation stone of human relationships. Highsmith, whether by instinct or design, situates her characters, Tom Ripley included, at strategic points where, however different the choices faced, they are always challenged both in relation to issues of good and evil, and as members of an ethical community. Drawing on Kant's notion of radical evil, ie. evil as a free choice, a product of human freedom, this chapter will look at how Highsmith's creation of her amoral anti-hero, who never gets caught or faces the moral consequences of his actions, allows her to approach issues such as proximity to others, human relationships and the limits of ethical behaviour.

Highsmith adored writing the Ripley novels: she turned to Ripley as a release from what she saw as her more depressing books, where her heroes, "are always chewing over their guilt, wondering how well they'll sleep at night with that on their conscience."[5] Ripley's appeal for her is that, "He's amoral about murder - he does it and then he reasons it away."[6] Yet the Ripley novels express a high level of anxiety, and critics argue that this is concerned with the numerous possibilities that his crimes may be discovered rather than any hint of an internal conscience:

> He reflects the amoral ego that all of us possess but few dare to recognise. Consequently he suffers no guilt, no remorse, only occasional twinges of doubt that his schemes (which start off simple and foolproof but escalate into catastrophic complication) may not work out quite right.[7]

The issue of the difference between guilt and anxiety is central here: the intense anxiety that pervades the Ripley novels is not merely due to a concern about getting caught. It is rather the device Highsmith uses to draw the reader in to a non-specific layer of unease that permeates every situation described, however peripheral to the main plot. Martin Heidegger argues that the difference between anxiety and fear (or guilt) is that anxiety is never about anything specific and in his words: "Anxiety reveals the Nothing. We 'hover' in anxiety. More precisely, anxiety leaves us hanging because it induces the slipping away of beings as a whole."[8]

Heidegger, in his analysis of anxiety, argues that it drives those who are affected by it to a position of distance from the world, where the sense of self is diminished and is experienced as a void: "Anxiety drains and this void cramps: the heart contracts. The external world becomes objectivized, rigidifies into lifelessness, and the inner self loses its centre of action, it depersonalizes itself. Anxiety is objectivization outside and depersonalization inside."[9] However, even Tom Ripley, often portrayed as Highsmith's exemplary monad, has to exist in a universe of other people; he works to illustrate the dangers and pitfalls of what Levinas terms 'proximity'; the "terrain of morality's most dazzling glory; but also of its most ignoble defeats."[10] Portraying how a contracted and rigidified Tom Ripley lives, in a universe of others, having to interrelate as a part of a society of human subjects, is one of the key elements of Highsmith's exploration of the treacherous terrain of the ethical relationship.

One of the most interesting aspects of Highsmith's work is the way in which she concentrates on the intricacies of her protagonist's obsessions with objects. This has led critics of her work to claim that she is uninterested in relationships between human beings. Russell Harrison, in *Patricia Highsmith* for example, believes that Highsmith's protagonists' fascination with objects actually underpins the texts, defining and giving meaning to the characters. In relation to Tom Ripley he argues:

> What constitutes the latent level of the novel is its fascination with objects, or what may be termed the novels *parti pris* for commodities, the objects that consumer society produces to be bought and possessed, which through such purchase and possession, serve to define their owner.[11]

Harrison continues to argue this point in respect of several of Highsmith's other 'heroes', claiming it to be a defining characteristic of both the form and content of her work. While she certainly exposes the myriad small obsessions with physical objects and ritual which structure everyday experience, her central concern is not with this in and for itself. Rather she uses objects as an anchor, as certainties in an uncertain and dangerous world where other people constitute a hazardous and ambivalent zone of experience.

In Kantian terms Tom Ripley treats other people as having 'value not dignity', in other words as having use value rather than, as Kant believed to constitute the moral and rational position, as ends in themselves. For Kant, human beings exist as rational members of what he terms a 'kingdom of ends', wherein universally valid laws constituted by human subjects, decree that persons must be treated as ends in themselves, rather than as objects, able to be used and discarded, or in other words as a means to an end. Kant constructed a system whereby the a priori part of ethics, known as the 'metaphysics of morals', and the experiential or empirical part, 'practical anthropology', cannot be confused if human beings are not to descend into what he termed 'moral degeneration'. For Kant, actions that can be classed as morally good have to be performed for the sake of duty alone, and only the a priori element of ethics is capable of showing us what duty is. If experience is taken into account then the pure impetus towards duty becomes contaminated with self-interest and the two, duty and self-interest, become confused. In Kant's schema, good will is and must be good in all circumstances and situations. Things that are good in many respects can and are classified as bad when used by a bad will. By positing this, Kant blocks all arguments based on the actual results of actions, arguing that a good situation can quite easily arise from actions taken for all the wrong, or bad, reasons.

The concept of duty is introduced to distinguish the good of an action, which for Kant, is the only criteria by which to judge whether an action has been carried out as a result of moral goodness or self interest.

One of Kant's formal maxims states that what gives moral worth to actions is doing one's duty for the sake of duty alone. For Kant this is a formal maxim, the content of the action is morally irrelevant, and whether or not the desired result actually occurs is similarly insignificant. This considered, the action is devoid of meaning outside the requirement to do one's duty regardless of self-interest.

Throughout his writing, and especially in 'Groundwork of the Metaphysic of Morals', Kant examines the strictures of the maxim that holds that man must act in good will, for the sake of duty alone. He develops the category of the categorical imperative, which states: "I ought never to act except in such a way *that I can also will that my maxim should become a universal law.*"[12] To make this clearer and to relate the first, very formal, statement of the categorical imperative to life experience, Kant adds two more formulas which he terms practical. The first prohibits using not just others, but one's own self, as means to an end: "*Act in such a way that you always treat humanity, whether in your own person or in the person of any other, never simply as a means, but always at the same time as an end.*"[13] The third formula relates the individual to other people as a member of a community, arguing that the categorical imperative, while necessarily concentrating on the 'I', also takes account of the primacy of intersubjectivity, relatedness to others:

> Reason thus related every maxim of the will, considered as making universal law, to every other will, and also to every action towards oneself: it does so, not because of any further motive or further advantage, but from the Idea of the *dignity* of a rational being who obeys no other law than that which he at the same time enacts himself.[14]

At this stage so far there doesn't seem to be much in Kant's philosophy to shed light on Highsmith's transgressive, self-interested and definitely non-dutiful hero. However, the categorical imperative, emphasising the necessity to treat the other person as an end never merely a means, is problematised in the text *Religion within the Limits of Reason Alone*. Here Kant develops the notion of radical evil, not theorised as a fact of nature but as a choice, a maxim as powerful as that outlined above: "Hence the source of evil cannot lie in an object *determining* the will through inclination, nor yet in a natural impulse; it can lie only in a rule made by the will for the use of its freedom, that is, in a maxim."[15]

The choice between a good and an evil maxim is, in Kant's argument a free act made depending on whether the moral law or sensuous nature predominates within each human being. Kant calls the propensity of the will to follow maxims which neglect the moral law, wickedness of the human heart, perversity and corruption, but refuses to separate the wicked man from the good, arguing instead that all human beings bear the possibility of evil within them.

The concept of radical evil was revolutionary in that it shifted the emphasis away from evil being viewed as diabolical or based on original sin. Prior to Kant's critical philosophy evil had been categorised as a deficit, something less tangible than 'good'. For him, evil is integral to human freedom, thus he shifts the debate into the arena of morality by asking why, given the fact of freedom, man might *choose* evil.

Highsmith was often taken to task for the manner in which Tom Ripley was able to perform acts regarded as evil, such as murder, for the sake of his self-interest, and then carry on a cultured, urbane existence without appearing different from others, albeit with a certain detachment and lack of conscience. The ways in which she illustrates this are never laboured; they emerge at certain points in the novels in the form of inappropriate or awkward responses that are quickly buried again as Ripley recognises that other people are unsettled by the differences between his responses and theirs. It seems that Highsmith was not criticised as much for the actions of her character, but rather for the fact that he gets away with them so well, unpunished by the Law in both the legal and psychoanalytic sense. She gives Ripley his own individual moral code: he almost exclusively abhors killing, gaining no vicarious pleasure from the act himself, viewing it instead as pure necessity. In this regard, he has nothing in common with the serial killer, drawn to the pleasure of the act of killing. He has no 'signature' marking his style of murder, instead his murders are radically instantaneous, erupting at often unforeseen moments when he concludes that all other avenues have been closed to him. Kant argues that radical evil is never evil for its own sake, for the sake of doing evil, but rather, as a force of will, is always in the service of self-interest. Ripley is hard to categorise as evil, he certainly performs evil actions, but at every crucial point throughout the novels he rationalises his actions - there is always a reason for what he does. While he can be read as amoral (and this is how Highsmith reads her creation) in actuality he never repudiates the moral law by stepping outside the boundaries of human relationships, ties of friendship or honour. In fact, the marriage of Tom and his wife Heloise, in its calm, almost ascetic simplicity, constitutes the most positive model of a human relationship anywhere in her work, where marriage or close contact with other people is usually portrayed as a vicious battleground.

The only times Ripley kills in a premeditated way are his

murders of Mafia members. Highsmith hated the Mafia and Ripley rationalises the murders of Mafia members by claiming that he is doing the world a service: "because the Mafia regard murder as man's way of proving himself."[16] For Tom Ripley, ridding the world of the vermin that he considered the Mafia to be, is entirely consistent with his moral code, and thus for him, becomes an ethical action. He regards reducing the effectiveness of the Mafia by murder, as his moral, disinterested duty.

Joan Copjec points out that Kant's redefinition of evil, "burdens us with full responsibility for our actions; we are no longer able to exonerate ourselves by claiming to be victims of our passions and thus of external circumstances."[17] The belief that evil was aligned with base, sensuous motives and good with man's will is shattered: the adoption of a good or an evil maxim becomes a radically free choice. In her account of radical evil she argues that Kant counters the historicist argument against his position by positing the inevitability of the bad outcome, locating in man, "a profound malignity that causes him to be bad even when he is good; that is, even as we heed the moral law, we do so, according to Kant, for self-interested reasons."[18]

Social circumstances enmesh man within a web of his failure to act disinterestedly, always seeking to elevate oneself in the eyes of the other, or as Lacan puts it: "man's desire finds its meaning in the desire of the other, not so much because the other holds the key to the object desired, as because the first object of desire is to be recognized by the other."[19] In *The Talented Mr. Ripley* Tom Ripley's first murder, the transgressive act that frees him to murder again and again with psychic impunity, is carried out primarily for reasons of self-interest, to gain financially and socially from the death. However, the moment in the novel that dismantles the barrier between fantasy and act itself, is crucially the point where Tom realises that Dickie does not recognise him, as he desires to be recognised:

> You were supposed to see the soul through the eyes, see love through the eyes, the one place you could look at another human being and see what really went on inside, and in Dickie's eyes Tom saw nothing more now than he would have seen if he had looked at the hard, bloodless surface of a mirror.[20]

At this point Ripley recognises the other person's irreconcilable difference but does not approach this as a responsibility, as proximity, a concept that: "stands for the unique quality of the ethical situation-which forgets reciprocity, as in love that does not expect to be shared"[21] Prior to this, he had begun to copy Dickie's gestures and mannerisms, in an attempt to get closer to him. While writing within a very different context, Jacques Derrida argues that proximity does not necessarily lead to empathy, indeed the closer the relationship, the greater the risk of the emergence of what Derrida terms 'unforgivable evil':

> There could be, in effect, all sorts of proximity (where the crime is between people who know each other): language, neighbourhood, familiarity, even family etc. But in order for evil to emerge, 'radical evil' and perhaps worse again, unforgivable evil, it is necessary that at the most intimate of that intimacy an absolute hatred would come to interrupt the peace. This destructive hostility can only aim at what Levinas calls the 'face' of the Other, the similar other, the closest neighbour, …within the same quarter, the same house, sometimes the same family.[22]

This is the pivotal turning point within the novel, when Ripley recognises the illusion of reciprocity:

> It struck Tom like a terrible truth, true for all time, true for all the people he had known in the past and for those he would know in the future: each had stood and would stand before him, and he would know time and time again that he would never know them, and the worst was that there would always be the illusion, for a time, that he did know them, and that they and he were completely in harmony and alike.[23]

Highsmith at this point tests the boundaries of morality by allowing her character complete understanding of his predicament: he then makes a free and clear choice for his forthcoming actions. Ripley, after his recognition of the schism between himself and other people, is then free to treat people, in Kant's terms, as having value not dignity. Throughout the rest of *The Talented Mr Ripley* Highsmith portrays Ripley as a loner, whose interaction with others is limited. When Ripley considers the pleasures that Dickie's money will bring him, these pleasures outweigh those of relating to other people: it is as if he has attempted to transpose the desire for the other's desire into the appropriation of objects and financial freedom that will allow him to avoid the illusion of harmony that he knows to be false. However, by the beginning of the second Ripley novel he is married and living, if not as part of a community, then at least on its fringes. He is able to sustain friendships, even if these are generally with people who are engaged in criminal activity with him. In fact Tom Ripley functions much more successfully than the tortured heroes of Highsmith's other novels, for whom the world becomes more and more alien and implosive. The difference between Tom Ripley and those around him, criminal or law abiding, is his lack of conscience or guilt.

Kant states that although transgressions of the moral law are impossible to avoid, man is always conscious of them, and they are never performed with a clear and easy heart: "No man who is not indifferent to morality can take pleasure in himself, can indeed escape a bitter dissatisfaction with himself, when he is conscious of maxims which do not agree with the moral law in him."[24] Radical evil is not elevated into a universal law; rather each act is felt as an exception to the way one *ought* to act. Joan Copjec links Kant's argument to Freud's notion of the superego, in that both posit the fundamental existence of guilt, which doesn't allow any of us, especially the most virtuous, off the hook:

> Saving his strongest denunciations for those acts that outwardly appear to be the most moral, Kant responds exactly like Freud's superego, which is most remorseless in its condemnation of precisely those who are the most conscientious about fulfilling their moral duty.[25]

The consequence of this argument is that man's guilt, or awareness of transgression, is the only way in which the law manifests itself to us. Copjec cites Lacan for a more contemporary way of putting it: "In Lacan's translation, the status of the subject becomes, with Kant, ethical rather than ontological; the subject can only be supposed on the basis of moral conscience."[26]

Patricia Highsmith's interest in the nature of guilt leads her to portray characters much given to introspection, whose desires and actions run contrary to their sense of right and wrong, and the ways in which they think they should behave. The Ripley novels, however, explore the contradictions inherent in a character amoral enough to commit murder but in other respects expressing a coherent moral code. Ripley transgresses the moral law through his acts of murder for self-interest, yet experiences no guilt for his actions and intentions. It is not that Ripley is unaware of the existence of the moral law, but he is able to elide the prohibition on murder by separating it from his own concept of morality. Highsmith contrasts her angst-ridden heroes' moral suffering with Ripley's foreclosure of guilt and emotion to expose and questions the ambiguities inherent in modern conceptions of morality, which prioritise uncertainty:

> The moral self moves, feels and acts in the context of ambivalence and is shot through with uncertainty. Hence the ambiguity-free moral situation has solely a utopian existence of the perhaps indispensable horizon and stimulus for a moral act, but not a realistic target of ethical practice.[27]

With her creation of a 'hero' who is so clearly not ambivalent about his actions and desires, Highsmith frees Ripley of all of the moral uncertainties that plague her other characters. I stated above that Tom Ripley despises murder. There is never any sense through these novels of a vicarious satisfaction at the carrying out of the act itself. Highsmith believed her main concern to be with the effects of guilt on her heroes. In some novels her heroes are guilty without charge from the very beginning, almost casting about for an action to 'fit' the level of guilt experienced. In the Ripley novels guilt is circumvented: if a sense of guilt correlates to the level of pleasure attained by carrying out an evil action, then Ripley's *lack* of pleasure could be seen to relate directly to his lack of guilt. Highsmith's suffering heroes do not enjoy their killings either, yet their moral codes trip them up nonetheless. By embracing a moral code that is flexible without being ambivalent, Ripley avoids Kant's 'ought' and the strictures of the superego.

The ways in which Highsmith's characters gain pleasures are complex and are never simply a straightforward enjoyment of the act itself. Contra Kant's notion of radical evil, Bataille argues that it is only the enjoyment of murder that makes it evil: "If a man kills for a material advantage his crime only really becomes a purely evil act if he actually enjoys committing it, independently of the advantage to be gained from it."[28] For Bataille then, enjoyment is the defining characteristic of the evil action. Throughout his work on evil Bataille does nevertheless argue that evil is transgressive, likening it to 'divine intoxication', caught within the instincts of childhood, yet at the same time closely aligned with a push towards death:

> Evil therefore, if we examine it closely, is not only the dream of the wicked: it is to some extent the dream of Good. Death is the punishment, sought and accepted for this mad dream, but nothing can prevent the dream from having been dreamt.[29]

So enjoyment becomes more complex than mere sadism, evil for the pleasure of the act alone.

Throughout Highsmith's novels the sense of intoxication is conveyed in several different ways. In the non-Ripley novels the chief protagonists are often either consumed by obsessions which culminate in suicide, choosing, in Bataille's sense, death as the inevitable consequence of the 'mad dream', or they are caught up in a Kafkaesque nightmare where they are surrounded by a spiralling madness that inevitably leads to death. In these cases the intoxication touches them, disrupts them, but they do not instigate it. While Highsmith's heroes in these novels are innocent in respect of the instigation of chaos, they are however, caught within its intoxicating consequences: they never convincingly try to extricate themselves from situations that are spiralling out of control. This is one of the ways that Highsmith builds up the tension and levels of anxiety that characterise her work: the point where we recognise that the hero is innocent yet guilty, caught in a nightmare yet, at some level, responsible.

Tom Ripley is exceptional in her work. He clearly and rationally chooses the evil act, not as a consequence of obsession but as a means to a particular end. He does however, exhibit the kind of anxiety highlighted by Heidegger, so that even while he avoids and seems to exist happily without guilt, a strong sense of anxiety pervades the texts. This anxiety, I would argue, imbues our reading of her work. She never interrupts the story with authorial intent, yet at the same time draws us into identifications with characters whose actions we would presumably never condone. Her seduction is to draw the reader in: "The reader has no choice but to follow the work, nothing could go another way. You are trapped in the very ease of reading. The result is like suffocation, losing breathe or will."[30]

If, as Kant argues, guilt is the only way to know the law then what does anxiety give knowledge of? Heidegger states that anxiety distances and induces the sense of reality to slip away, shifting a sense of self into a void of nothingness. In her portrayal of Ripley, Highsmith presents the reader with a character who freely chooses the evil action, feels no guilt at this choice, and recognises the illusion of reciprocity. If radical evil allows the possibility of treating others as means not ends, it could be argued that through anxiety Ripley distances himself from the consequences of this choice, while at the same time diminishing experience and relationships with others to a level of depersonalisation and objectification.

In his book *Job and the Excess of Evil*, Philippe Nemo shifts the problem of evil back to the *Book of Job*, a text traditionally considered problematic within the framework of the Bible.[31] According to Nemo, the

Book of Job introduces the idea of evil as a shifting construct that cannot be attached to something external but has to be addressed as the 'why me?' - a lament incidentally which occurs in many of Highsmith's texts, including the Ripley novels. *The Book of Job* ends in a resolution between Job and God as he turns away from the Devil, but as Richard Kearney points out, the text is an exemplary example of the attempt to make moral sense of out what is chaotic and unspeakable precisely by engaging in dialogue:

> The wisdom genre turns lament into a legal complaint. It tries to make moral sense out of the monstrous …With such wisdom literature; the enigma of evil becomes less a matter of metaphysical giveness than of interpersonal relations (human-human or human-divine).[32]

Nemo argues that the Book of Job says:

> the excess of evil does indeed destroy the world, yet not in order to reveal another "world" - an inverted image of this one caught in a co-eternal, and eternally futile, struggle with it - but to reveal what is *other* than the world, that is to say, what is other than worldliness as such, other than the neutral legality of the world.[33]

What is revealed by this excess, he argues, is the soul but not as part of the ordered legality of the world, but *in waiting*, subject to, but not contained by, the Law or in Job's case, by God: "For his vision of a soul *in waiting* is not the commentary to a vague conviction: it is the interpretation of the very phenomenon of evil, inasmuch as evil is in excess."[34]

In Job's case, the discourse of the soul in waiting is with God. If we strip the religious elements from it, it becomes a soul in waiting for death, in Heidegger's sense, but paradoxically at the same time a soul waiting to exist, yet barred by anxiety from experiencing life other than through the screen of evil. For Bataille evil is intertwined with death yet is at the same time, similar to the Freudian idea of the death drive, a basis of existence: "Since death is the condition of life, Evil, which is essentially cognate with death, is also, in a somewhat ambiguous manner, a basis of existence."[35] Levinas, in his response to Nemo's text, argues: "Anxiety is the sharp point at the heart of evil"[36], and that evil lived as suffering is revealed though the experience of anxiety:

> In agreement with Heidegger, anxiety is interpreted as a

discourse of nothingness, as being-towards death, as the
fact of a world that sneaks away and isolates man, and
the fact of a human being who closes himself off to
words of consolation that still belong to the resources of
this sneaking world.[37]

The worlds in which Highsmith situates her characters range
from exemplary examples of that 'ordered legality' that her heroes are
subject to, but not contained by, to sites of chaos with unfamiliar and
confusing rules which mock any semblance of order. Highsmith does not
write detective fiction, and the representation of the Law within her work,
in the guise of the police, never performs the function of containment. In
other words the Law does not capture the excesses of her protagonists,
whether or not they are eventually caught for their crimes. There is a sense
in Highsmith that the Law operates on some different, simpler level to that
of her protagonists: that while the police are concerned with the simple
facts of the case, and often blunder their way to the wrong conclusion
about even that, her engagement is with something else.
     While the presence of the police is a factor throughout most of
Highsmith's novels, they generally function to illustrate their irrelevance
to the deeper issues that she is concerned with. Her protagonists may be,
and often are, anxious about their legal culpability for crimes committed,
and in Tom Ripley's case spend much of the novels dodging discovery,
but this is merely the device utilised by Highsmith to draw the reader in
towards the underlying dimension of anxiety described by Levinas above.
     Reviewers have often found Highsmith's work fascinating if
problematic as crime fiction due to the difficulty of grasping, through
seemingly accessible prose, the meaning or intentionality behind her
stories.[38] Characters such as Tom Ripley are isolated in Levinas's sense,
closed off to words both of consolation or compassion and used by
Highsmith to nudge at the boundaries of legality through the use of the
medium of crime fiction with its assumptions of good and bad. Their
anxiety, whether we interpret it as 'disclosure of nothingness', or 'being-
towards death', which as Levinas says gives access to the heart of evil,
disallows them from completely joining the worlds in which Highsmith
insists on situating them.
     Highsmith never allows the reader to get comfortable with her
work. A sense of discomfort pervades both her characters and their
situations, arguably most effectively in the Ripley novels. The unease built
up through the Ripley texts gradually distances him from the world, even
as he appears to become part of it through ritual and the dependence on
objects. The offer of stability, or normality, is often forthcoming but is

never able to be accepted. According to Levinas, this disturbance is
characteristic of evil as excess:

> In evil's appearing, in its original phenomenality, in its
> *quality*, there is announced a *modality*, a manner: the
> not-finding-a-place, the refusal to be comfortable with
> … a counter-nature, a monstrosity, the of-itself
> disturbing and alien.[39]

Nemo categorises the truth of evil as the inability of the subject who is
caught within this excess to be able to become free of it: "The truth of evil
discloses itself precisely in not allowing the individual who is caught in its
vertigo to exit the vertigo and join the world in its stability."[40]

Heidegger's distinction between anxiety and guilt (or fear as he
terms it) based on the argument that anxiety is objectless, is disputed by
Jacques Lacan, who believes rather that while anxiety does not have a
specific cause, it does however have an object. Alenka Zupancic, in her
reading of Kant and Lacan from the questioning perspective of ethics,
points out that, for Lacan: "anxiety is not a 'subjective' but, rather, an
'objective' feeling. It is a *'feeling that does not deceive'* (Lacan), one
which indicates that we have come near to the 'object'."[41] For Lacan, the
idea that there is no object of anxiety can lead to a denial of the reality of
what might threaten us. Approached through this perspective, Tom
Ripley's 'contraction of the heart' and seemingly aimless anxiety would
work as a protective device; rather than causing him to 'slip away' in
Heidegger's sense: it may be his only anchor in a non-reciprocal universe.

The argument that anxiety is not objectless does not however lead
to a belief in the self-evidence of evil. Zupancic argues that evil
structurally constitutes a void that can never be fully represented. She uses
literary texts to illustrate the ways in which evil, in order to function as
evil, must be placed at a point of non-comprehension, for which there can
be no explanation, no beyond: "In these stories, as well as in what
constitutes the individual or the collective Imaginary, evil is usually
precisely this: that which lends its 'face' to some disturbing void 'beyond
representation'."[42] According to Zupancic, within stories that play on the
contrast between 'good' and 'evil' characters, the reader's fascination is
for the 'evil' character. Not a revolutionary idea, but the often cited reason
for this is that the 'evil' character is somehow 'deeper' than the 'good'
character, who may be viewed as one-dimensional or flat. She argues that
this explanation is not adequate in that: "the moment we get any kind of
psychological or other explanation for why somebody is 'evil', the spell is
broken, so to speak."[43]

While Highsmith offers tantalising clues into Tom Ripley's background there is never any sense that these 'explain' his actions or account for his difference from others. Highsmith was criticised for the 'flatness' of her prose and the ways in which her characters simply act, without in-depth analysis of their situations. Ripley is the prime example of this. He may gain no pleasure from the act of murder, but in *Ripley's Game* he causes murders to happen for the fun of it, because he is bored. Zupancic contends that the perceived complexity of 'evil' characters lies in the fact that there is no adequate explanation for what they do, other than, "the fun (or spite) of it. In this sense they are as 'flat' as can be. But at the same time, this lack of depth can itself become something palpable, a most oppressive and massive presence."[44]

Zupancic's reading connects the 'oppressive and massive presence' which is based on lack rather than a tangible substance, to the ways in which evil manages to capture the imagination, repulsive yet fascinating at the same time: "Fascination could be said to be the aesthetic feeling of contradiction ... 'Evil' is not only something we abhor more than anything else; it is also something that manages to catch hold of our desire."[45] In Lacanian psychoanalytic terms, she argues that evil and the Imaginary are linked in that evil has no image while: "the Imaginary register is in itself a response to the lack of the Image."[46]

This psychoanalytical insight is useful for an analysis of evil within literary texts, in that it addresses issues of why evil fascinates and how that fascination is produced and perpetuated. Zupancic argues that it is precisely because of evil's lack of substance, for example in stories where the evil characters are perceived to be deeper than they actually are, where we as readers, search for the 'meaning' of the character, that a multiplicity of attempts to imagine evil can be produced and remain endlessly fascinating:

> The more this lack or absence is burdensome, the more frenetic is the production of images ... the more closely an image gets to occupy the very place of the lack of the Image, the greater will be its power of fascination.[47]

Zupancic explains that in Lacan's theory of the construction of the human subject, there occurs a symbolically designated "place of the lack of the image". Therefore, due to the mechanics of representation, a designated 'beyond representation' is generated. This is generally viewed as transgressive and often, according to Zupancic, evil in that it cannot be encompassed within the dual parameters of the Imaginary and the Symbolic. Every image produced to represent this 'evil' is therefore opposite to its effect: "The point is not that real evil cannot be illustrated or represented, but that we have a tendency to call 'evil' precisely that which is not represented in a given representation."[48] In this sense Zupancic designates evil as an effect of the Real: "the last veil or 'screen' that separates us from the impossible Real."[49]

Through these arguments Zupancic comes to the conclusion that evil can be said to occupy the place of the impossible, yet argues that 'the impossible' is also the space of ethics. Turning to Kant's theory of radical evil to support her, she argues that Kant recognised that the good, exemplified by the categorical imperative, has no other content apart from the universality of the moral law. As already explained, the only reason to obey the moral law, according to Kant, is for its own sake and with no other motive, all other motives implying self-interest. Zupancic argues that Kant's total insistence on adherence to the moral law *for its own sake* bleeds the concept of all content. Since there is no content, the moral law becomes something that the human being cannot in fact transgress: "One can fail to act 'according to the principle and only out of the principle' but this failure cannot be called a transgression."[50]

There are many examples in which Kant's moral law could be followed for purely 'legal' (ie. performed in accordance with the law) but not 'ethical' or 'good' (by which Kant means those acts which are performed only because of the moral law and for no other reason). Therefore, according to Zupancic, it is possible to become 'radically evil' while keeping within the letter of the law: "A radically evil man is not someone whose only motive is to do 'bad things', or someone who couldn't care less about the law. It is rather someone who willingly conforms to the law, provided he can get the slightest benefit out of it."[51]

Tom Ripley is capable of conforming both to the moral and external law, provided he can get some benefit from it. He never descends into what Kant terms 'diabolical evil', where evil is elevated into a maxim which opposes the moral law on every occasion. Here, evil becomes an 'incentive of the will', where the subject acts contrary to the moral law, even if those actions threaten or oppose his own self interests. Evil thus becomes a 'duty' in the same sense as 'good will', even if it leads to the death or destruction of the subject.

For Tom Ripley, evil is never a duty in the sense of diabolical evil; instead it arises from both self-interest and what he perceives as unsavoury necessity. The central preoccupation of the Ripley novels lies in Tom Ripley's attempts at self-preservation, both as 'law-abiding citizen' and as author of his own moral code. Whether we read the anxiety that assails him as objectless or, in Lacan's sense, his *feeling that does not deceive* which may function to ensure the preservation of his 'self',

Highsmith has created with Ripley, a character exemplary in revealing the possibility of evil in a radical rather than a diabolical sense.

Once Ripley recognises the limits of proximity he is able to act for his own benefit, disregarding the status of the other person. Highsmith cleverly situates him within both a marriage and a community, forcing an uncomfortable juxtaposition between the outsider who finds it easier to relate to objects than other people, and husband, friend and business associate, for whom interaction is essential. Thereby she is able to foreground the difficulties faced by the contracted heart who, at some level, recognises yet cannot escape from, his isolation. Tom Ripley's attempts to 'stabilise' his world through imposing order and aestheticism on his surroundings, represent her most poignant reminders of his inability to break free of the excess of evil that captivates both him, and Highsmith's readers.

Notes

1. Highsmith, 1974 , 443.
2. Manvell, 1977, 23 - 24. Highsmith Archive.
3. 'Berlindale', 1968, 46 - 48. February. Highsmith Archive
4. Symons, 1964, 67. Highsmith Archive.
5. Herbert, 1974, 73. Highsmith Archive.
6. Ibid.
7. Meek, 1977, 33. Highsmith Archive.
8. Heidegger, 1977, 101.
9. Safranski, 1998, 179.
10. Bauman,1993, 87.
11. Harrison, 1997, 26.
12. Kant, 1948, 67.
13. Ibid. p. 91.
14. Ibid. p. 96.
15. Kant, 1960, p17.
16. Cosgrave, 1974, 46. Highsmith Archive.
17. Copjec, 1996, xi.
18. Ibid.
19. Lacan, 1977, 58.
20. Highsmith, 1955, 71.
21. Bauman, 87.
22. Derrida, 2001, 51.
23. Highsmith, 1955, 71.
24. Kant, 1960, 41.
25. Copjec, 1996, xiv.

26. Ibid., xv.
27. Bauman, 11.
28. Bataille, 1973, 18.
29. Ibid. 21.
30. Weinstein, 1982, 26. Highsmith Archive.
31. "The Book of Job, we read in certain Christian interpretations, is 'disconcerting', if not 'repulsive'. After such a first statement, one expects these exegetes to throw in the towel and file the text of Job away - and the text must be very strange indeed in the eyes of their doctrines - under the category of radical interrogation. Yet they make nothing of it". Nemo, 1998, 3.
32. Kearney, 2001, 107.
33. Nemo, 2.
34. Ibid., 3.
35. Bataille, 29.
36. Immanuel Levinas, 'Transcendence and Evil', in Nemo, 171.
37. Ibid.
38. "Her subjects' state of mind is affected by a kind of creeping airlessness. The same can be said of her prose, which registers every action - violent or not - in the same matter-of-fact way, so that the reader's sense of perspective becomes that of a Seeing Eye Dog." Clapp, 1999, Highsmith Archive.
39. Levinas, 'Transcendence and Evil', in Nemo, 1998, 173.
40. Nemo, 40.
41. Zupancic, 2000, 145.
42. Zupancic, 2001, 76.
43. Ibid.
44. Ibid.
45. Ibid., 75.
46. Ibid.
47. Ibid.
48. Ibid.
49. Ibid., 76.
50. Ibid.
51. Ibid., 79.

References

Bataille, G. (1973), *Literature and Evil*. A. Hamilton (trans). London and New York: Marion Boyars.

Bauman, Z. (1993), *Postmodern Ethics*. Oxford: Blackwell.

'Berlindale', (1968), February. Highsmith Archive.

Clapp, S. (1999), 'The Simple Act of Murder', *The New Yorker*, Dec. 20th. Highsmith Archive. 16

Copjec, J. (ed) (1996), *Radical Evil*. London: Verso.

Cosgrave, P. (1974), 'Crime Compendium'. *The Spectator*. 23rd March. Highsmith Archive. 46-48

Derrida, J. (2001), *On Cosmopolitanism and Forgiveness*. M. Dooley and M. Hughes (trans). London: Routledge.

Heidegger, M. (1977) 'What is Metaphysics?', in: *Martin Heidegger: Basic Writings*. D. Farrell Krell (ed.). San Francisco: Harper and Row.

Harrison, R. (1997), *Patricia Highsmith*. New York: Twayne.

Herbert, H. (1974), 'Maid a Killing'. *Arts Guardian*. 18th March. Highsmith Archive. 73

Highsmith, P. (1974), *Ripley's Game*. In the collection *The Mysterious Mr. Ripley*. London: Penguin.

Highsmith, (1955), *The Talented Mr. Ripley*. In the collection *The Mysterious Mr. Ripley*. London, Penguin.

Hitchcock. A. (director) (1951), *Strangers on a Train*. [film]. Warner Bros. USA.

Kant, (1948), 'Groundwork of the Metaphysic of Morals', in: H.J. Paton (ed.) *The Moral Law,* London: Hutchinson.

Kant, (1960), *Religion Within the Limits of Reason Alone*, Theodore M.Greene and Hoyt H.Hudson (eds.). New York: Harper and Row.

Kearney, R. (2001), 'Others and Aliens', in: J. L. Geddes (ed.). *Evil After Postmodernism*. London: Routledge. 107.

Lacan, J. (1977), 'Function and Field of Speech and Language', in: A.

Sheridan (trans). *Ecrits*, London: Tavistock. 30-109

Manvell, R. (1977), *British Book News*, pages 23-24. August. In Highsmith Archive, Swiss National Library. Bern, Switzerland.

Meek, S. (1977),'Patricia Highsmith'. *Time Out*. January. Highsmith Archive. 33-34

Minghella, A. (director) (1999). *The Talented Mr. Ripley* [film]. Miramax Films. USA.

Nemo, P. (1998), *Job and the Excess of Evil*. M. Kigel (trans) with a postscript by E. Levinas. Pittsburgh: Duquesne University Press.

Safranski, R. (1998), *Martin Heidegger; Beyond Good and Evil*. E. Osers (trans). Cambridge: Harvard University Press.

Symons, J. (1964), 'Terror all the Way'. *Sunday Times*. 23rd February. Highsmith Archive. 67

Weinstein, J. (1982), 'The Case of the Misplaced Author'. *Village Voice Supplement*. August. Highsmith Archive. 26

Zupancic, A. (2000), *Ethics of the Real*. London: Verso.

Zupancic, A. (2001), 'On Evil: An interview With Alenka Zupancic'. *Cabinet,* Winter: 5. New York: Immaterial Incorporated. 74-79

"I did so many bad things": Sin and Redemption in the Films of Abel Ferrara

Paul Davies

I am in search of some kind of truth according to God. I know I didn't create the universe. Someone else did. So I'm in that search.

Abel Ferrara

Abel Ferrara is best known for his violent exploitation films and powerfully intense and brutal portraits of New York's mean streets. Having started off as an independent filmmaker, his reputation has since widened beyond a mere cult audience. What perhaps surprisingly links all his films is a serious, at times searingly honest attempt to deal with religious themes. It is hardly surprising then, that the critical reception of Ferrara's films was at first marked by initial confusion and rejection, much of which was stirred up by censorship and 'video nasties' controversies, particularly concerning *The Driller Killer* and *Bad Lieutenant*, and by the feeling that Ferrara was nothing more than a cheap slasher-cum-porno monger. With time such uncritical, vituperative abuse subsided and a more sober, serious tone took over reflected by six book-length studies with a seventh upcoming, in addition to articles in the British film journal *Sight and Sound* and the International Abel Ferrara Internet Library, by far the most comprehensive reference guide to all things Ferrara.[1]

Studies by Nick Johnstone and Bernd Kiefer/Marcus Stiglegger are likely to remain standard for some time. Although marred by an approach that mostly does nothing more than retell the content of the films, Johnstone's *Abel Ferrara: The King of New York* nevertheless manages a close enough reading of Ferrara's work and establishes relevant connections between the films. Though symptomatic of the author's determinedly biographical orientation, the thirty-six page introduction entitled "Notes on Ferrara", does unearth important aspects of the director's life and approach to film making, and Johnstone must be given due credit in two areas. First, he acknowledges the crucial role of religion in Ferrara's oeuvre, something too many critics are still reluctant to do, believing instead that Ferrara merely (mis)uses Catholic symbols and iconography for his own ends - whatever they are. Second, Johnstone recognizes the key contributions of Ferrara's close circle of regular collaborators as well as his status as a genuine *auteur* whose influences include Pasolini, Godard, Bresson, Polanski and Fassbinder. More scholarly by far however, is the book by the two German academics Bernd Kiefer and Marcus Stiglegger. Entitled *Die bizarre Schönheit der Verdammten: Die Filme von Abel Ferrara* (*The bizarre beauty of the damned: The films of Abel Ferrara*). This work contains an introductory essay by the two editors on Ferrara's search for redemption - like Johnstone, the authors have no trouble identifying Ferrara as a filmmaker with deeply spiritual and religious concerns who is fascinated by definitions of good and evil - along with eight other contributions which deal with issues ranging from sex(uality), death and an interpretation of Ferrara's protagonists in the light of Kierkegaard's work, to Ferrara as a director of 'neo-Noirs,' his filmic topography of New York, the role of Rap and Hip Hop on his soundtracks, and a welcome in-depth analysis of *New Rose Hotel*. The book as a whole and the introductory essay in particular, come to the conclusion that Ferrara's central theme, present from the very beginning, is the violence of the infernal world of the city in which his protagonists more and more desperately search for redemption.[2]

The aim of this chapter is to demonstrate how many of the characters in Abel Ferrara's films face quasi-religious moral dilemmas revolving around questions of sin and redemption. They experience a descent into violence, often provoked by a desire for revenge which then turns into a voyage of self-discovery before resolving itself in the discovery of some sort of inner, often spiritual truth. Above all, Ferrara's films force us to decide how to face up to the implications of our often violent actions and to take responsibility for them.

Although Ferrara constantly, almost obsessively, returns to the same themes, I would nevertheless like to analyse the director's films in three sections, which progress chronologically throughout his oeuvre, in order to determine whether any thematic developments take place after all. In the first I will look at those films Ferrara made before *The King of New York* which have a desire for some sort of revenge as a central theme. In section two I will deal with what I believe are the four key Ferrara films in three thematically connected groups rather than in a strictly chronological order: (i) *King of New York* (1990), which shows the devastating effects of violence, murder and the lack of a spiritual anchor; (ii) *The Funeral* (1996), in which the characters justify their actions by recourse to a form of Catholicism which is not only the bleakest form possible, but which also misinterprets the concept of grace; (iii) the films *Bad Lieutenant* (1992) and *The Addiction* (1994) both of which offer much more concrete solutions to the problems of evil and human wickedness in terms of faith. So what we have here is a sort of sliding scale from ignorance to misguidedness to final enlightenment. Section three will briefly cover the work Ferrara has done in the last five years or so since *The Funeral*. I will then draw some conclusions on the Ferrara phenomenon and try to articulate the links between his films.[3]

1.   Aftershocks

As a teenager during the 1970s, Abel Ferrara started making short amateur films on Super 8 and inexpensive movies in New York which were expressions of an anti-Vietnam stance.[4] Ferrara shot these films together with a close group of friends many of whom are still colleagues, above all his long-term collaborator Nicholas St. John, who to date has written the screenplays for ten of Ferrara's films.[5] Ferrara directed his first real commercial film, *The Driller Killer* in 1979.[6] The narrative follows Lower East Side painter Reno Miller, played by the director himself under the pseudonym Jimmy Laine, who after being driven crazy by a punk band practicing in the apartment next to his, radically redirects his creative impulses by going on a killing spree with a Black and Decker. This was the first Ferrara film in which the issue of violence played a key role as it did in the film that followed two years later *Ms. 45*, with the appropriate alternative title of *Angel of Vengeance*. Often regarded by critics as a feminist reworking of the vigilante topos of films such as the *Death Wish* series, it is the story of Thana, a mute worker in New York's garment district who is raped twice in one day. At first traumatized and then driven over the edge by this horrendous experience, she undertakes an orgy of vengeance against the city's predatory males armed with the eponymous .45.

Both *The Driller Killer* and *Ms. 45* feature lead characters who decide to take the law into their own hands in order to exact vengeance. In *Fear City* the same theme is doubled. On the one hand we have the psychopathic serial slasher/killer Pazza, who ritualistically attacks, maims and murders female strippers in Manhattan. On the other there is the ex-boxer Matt Rossi, who runs the Starlite Agency booking company that provides the strip joints with strippers. Pazza believes he can disregard the law because he is so strong and perfect. In fact, as we hear in voice-over he is seeking to attain ultimate perfection: "With the death of each criminal, each whore, each worthless life, man comes closer to purity."[7] Pazza is a narcissistic loner whose self-absorption even comes out in his fighting style, a bizarre mixture of karate and kickboxing which is there not only to torture and prolong the agony of his victims, but to enable him to show off and play to the gallery as well - his own private gallery.

Pazza is paired off against Rossi. Whereas Pazza is a masculinist, body-building individualist striving for perfection, Rossi is embedded in the community of his booking company, feminized through his dealings with the women who closely surround him (not to mention the way the actor Tom Berenger is lit along with his distinctly 'feminine' appearance and performance) and flawed, even possibly fallen, since he accidentally killed his opponent in the ring some years ago, retiring from boxing as a result. The alleyway confrontation between Pazza and Rossi brings this contrast to a climax. The main reason Rossi is able to defeat his opponent is that Pazza loses himself in his self-absorbed, ritualistic posturing. Rossi's straightforward boxing style is ultimately more effective because he practices and trains with others, in contrast to the serial killer's self-made, self-trained regimen, which is more concerned with finely honed muscles and only really effective when surprising helpless victims. After all, the sole sparring partner Pazza has is himself, as we see in the scene where he kickboxes his own reflection in a mirror.

   Fear City also deals with the question of the remission of sins, and it is here that we see in embryo a theme that will fully emerge in Ferrara's later films. By confronting Pazza, Rossi simultaneously comes face to face with his own past as a boxer. In a confessional he asks a priest whether he can be forgiven in advance for a sin he is about to commit. The priest replies that he should first ask God's forgiveness for having offended him: "You can withhold it from me, but not the Lord. Ask for his guidance in this matter and let us recite the act of contrition together." So in *Fear City* we can witness the first inklings of the future Ferrara dichotomy between ruthless, individualist, unforgiving Protestantism and a more community-oriented, forgiving Catholicism that was to resurface in parts of *Bad Lieutenant* and which is the main concern of *The Addiction*.

   A further indication that Ferrara was by now moving in this direction is provided by *The Gladiator* (1986). Though a minor telemovie shot in two weeks and based on a television story and screenplay by William Bleich (with no Ferrara/St. John input) it still has the most important Ferrara hallmarks of his mid-80s films, namely the themes of vengeance and forgiveness. Master mechanic Rick Benton, loses his brother to a homicidal maniac who kills motorists at random in his "death car." After a run-in with a gang of punks who destroy his truck, Benton decides to become another of Ferrara's vigilantes and to this end converts his pick-up into a dangerous armed vehicle. Hunting down reckless drivers, Benton nevertheless leaves them alive and handcuffed for the police to find. At one point he offers a possible explanation for his behaviour: "Sometimes you think you're doing the right thing and it screws up. Everything goes wrong and you get in so deep that you can't get yourself out of it. You just can't stop." After this 'confession' Benton does eventually exact revenge and kill, "the guy who killed my brother. The Gladiator is finished." He is no longer at odds with himself.[8]

2.   Finding Enlightenment

As I mentioned earlier, in this section of Ferrara's films we can witness how his protagonists move from ignorance to misguidedness to enlightenment. First of all, we have *King of New York*. Ruthless drug lord Frank White has just been released from prison. At a party to celebrate his release he proclaims he is "back from the dead," and later at dinner in a restaurant maintains he has "been reformed." Resurrection and a chance to redeem himself? Hardly. At the same party he confesses he feels "no remorse" and then adds with an ironic laugh "and it's a terrible thing." Soon enough, White gets back into his role as a big time gangster and sets out to become 'King of New York' by gaining control of a multiracial gang of drug dealers. However, he claims he is now a man with a vision who feels bad about the way he has lived his life up to now: "If I can have a year or two," he tells his girlfriend, "I'll make something good." The purpose he has since found is to spin off some of the profits from his drug trade to finance a hospital for underprivileged children in the South Bronx which the government can't afford: "Why should all the hospitals be in the rich neighbourhoods?" asks White, which if he weren't a criminal would otherwise be completely valid.

Yet we must never forget that at the same time White is a walking contradiction. His drug-dealing hirelings are busy eliminating the competitors to enable his rise to the top of the crime lords in the city. And while White definitely does want to help out the less fortunate, he is not above doing harm to those very same people in the process. Neither can any of this be excused by the fact that on the other hand it's the police who are portrayed as the vigilantes in the film who have to break the law to achieve their aim of putting White away for life. Without a coherent spiritual and theological vision that tries to tackle one of the most fundamental of human problems, namely the existence of evil and injustice in the world, someone like White is caught in a contradictory position from which there is no way out, and which ultimately reveals him to be at best a misguided idealist or "confused moralist" and at worst a self-seeking hypocrite.[9] While trying to justify his actions to detective Bishop, his main adversary, in another of Ferrara's 'confessional' scenes, White argues that he has "never killed anyone that didn't deserve it." Bishop then asks him: "Who made you judge and jury?" White's seemingly cold-hearted response that, "Well, it's a tough job, but someone's gotta do it" is however, undercut by the tears which start to well up in his eyes. When he is then fatally wounded by Bishop towards the end of the film, White's "I don't need forever" emerges as a recognition that he has wasted his chance of a genuine new beginning.

The Funeral is a meditation on the dark certainty that violence begets violence. In 1930s New York, an Italian American family mourns the murder of Johnny Tempio. As he lies in his coffin, his grieving, furious brothers Ray and Chez are inextricably caught in a cycle of brutality in which vengeance is the only available option. Through a childhood memory of Ray's, we see why. Taking his three sons into a warehouse, the unseen Tempio patriarch shows Ray, Chez and Johnny a captured enemy who has dishonoured the family. Compassion is one thing, Ray's father tells him, but if this captive is set free, he's bound to kill them all, driven by the fear that the Tempios might change their minds about letting him live. The old man hands Ray a gun and tells him to execute the prisoner. Obsessed with finding and killing his brother's murderer, Ray finds himself in a grim replay of that very traumatic, childhood experience.

The family's Catholic faith can't help them at all here as their priest realizes when he says that, "the only way anything is going to change is if this family has a total reversal", and he goes on to lecture Ray's wife about the "practical atheism" her family lives every day. The main reason their faith cannot help them, is because they are labouring under a fundamental misconception concerning the nature of Catholic grace. This becomes clear in the following exchange between Ray and his wife Jean on the front porch of their two-storey house:

> RAY: If I do something wrong, it's because God didn't give me the grace to do what's right. Nothing happens without His permission. So if this world stinks, it's His fault. I'm only working with what I've been given.
> JEAN: So, that way, the people they found with bullet holes in their skulls, they're God's fault? Aren't you ashamed of yourself?
> RAY: I'm ashamed of nothing. I didn't make the world.
> JEAN: But you're not doing anything to make it better.
> RAY: Yeah, and I'll roast in Hell.

The practical implications of this wrong-headed point of view are horrendous. In one scene an axe-wielding Ray considers killing a character he knows didn't really deserve to die and arrives at what for him is a logical conclusion: "Since you're never going to forget this - you leave me no choice." The victim is therefore doomed not for what he did, but because of what Ray has done in response to it. This really is a sort of gruesome Calvinist 'inevitable damnation' theology run wild with no room whatsoever for forgiveness and the possibility that we can actually change our natures and make peace with God. This is the context in which a comment by Ferrara should be considered. He once said that his idea of redemption was, "I just don't wanna walk out of here having fucked somebody around, or have someone suffer for the fact I was on earth" as Ray makes his victim suffer in *The Funeral*.[10]

3.   The Redemption of Catholicism

Personal self-confrontation and a re-evaluation lie at the heart of the next two Ferrara films under discussion. Ferrara's fascination with the depths to which the human soul is capable of plummeting and the belief in the redemptive power of Catholicism, find their most potent expression in *Bad Lieutenant* and *The Addiction*.

At the centre of *Bad Lieutenant* is a corrupt and depraved New York police lieutenant referred to only as Lt. Hooked on drugs, alcohol and gambling, he is offered a material way out in the form of a $50,000 reward to find the two men guilty of a particularly heinous crime: they raped a nun on a church altar, using a crucifix and leaving the word 'fuck' written in graffiti on the altar as a sign of their scornful contempt. In this same church, the nun now tells Lt. she has forgiven her torturers. She obviously doesn't want the crime avenged like he does, and the lieutenant wonders how she can do this and whether she has the right to let the culprits go since her forgiveness could lead to other women being raped. She replies: "Talk to Jesus, pray ... He died for our sins."

The nun leaves the church after having pressed her rosary into Lt.'s hands, and the lieutenant then has a vision of Jesus Christ after his crucifixion. This vision will now be described in some detail because along with the finale to *The Addiction* it is *the* prime example of a Ferrara epiphany. Alone before the altar, Lt. starts to howl, moan, and whimper. He throws the rosary at the Christ figure and accuses him amongst other things of complete inactivity in the face of human suffering, a classic accusation throughout the ages:

> Is there something you wanna say to me, you fuck? What? Say something. Just don't stand there. What am I gonna do? You've gotta say something. You fuck, you fucking stand there and want me to do every fucking thing. Where were you? Where the fuck were you? I did so many bad things. I'm sorry. I'm weak. I tried, but I'm too fucking weak. Help me! Why didn't you help me? Forgive me! Forgive me, father, please!

He drops to his knees and crawls, if not downright grovels, on all fours towards his vision of Christ, who looks down at Lt. and offers him his right hand. As the lieutenant kisses his bloodied feet, he looks up and sees an elderly black woman in front of him holding the communion cup that the two culprits stole. The woman then leads the Lt. to the rapists.

The vision of Christ transforming into one of the locals demonstrates that the lieutenant is capable of emerging from his shell after all and establishing some sort of bond with other people. A self-destructive egocentric incapable of communication and totally isolated from the outside world as a result, he has now discovered love and compassion for his fellow women and men. His subsequent actions show strength and the influence Jesus can have on our lives, thereby proving that Christ has not been inactive as the lieutenant claimed. In fact, Lt. has been called a Christ figure because he takes on the suffering of the world and forgives sinners and rapists: certainly the lieutenant's crawl toward the Christ figure, in his own version of the stations of the cross in the sequence I just described, would back up such a reading.[11] Once Lt. finds the culprits, he gives them a second chance and money to start a new existence in another town. And even though he ends the film still strung out, washed out, and eventually shot and killed, this act of forgiveness redeems him. This contrast to the redemption denied to White in *King of New York* and Chez and Ray at the end of *The Funeral*, couldn't be more stark. As Harvey Keitel himself put it concerning his role: "The lieutenant has a deep need. He's a family man; he has children. He knows he is bad. He has a deep need for redemption."[12]

In many ways *The Addiction* replays the scenario of *Bad Lieutenant* with philosophy doctoral student Kathleen Conklin (as the lieutenant figure) similarly descending into vileness before finding salvation. But the film goes beyond *Bad Lieutenant* by attacking some of the essential views of evil in Protestant Calvinism. *The Addiction* was not exactly released to critical acclaim in 1994. This negative response however, was based on a fundamental misreading of the text. On a first viewing, it seems that by succumbing to vampiric urges, Conklin is better able to understand the vampire as a mirror of the cruelty of human history. Vampires therefore emerge as metaphors for an evil endemic to all of us. The film invites us to see them as undead because 'evil never dies': in classical vampire lore, vampires cannot look in a mirror as they reflect the raw, exposed face of evil. On this level, the film acts as a meditation on whether or not human nature has a fundamental predisposition toward committing depraved acts: this is reinforced through images of massacres in Vietnam and the Holocaust. In the opening sequence, Conklin leaves a Holocaust museum and debates the point of convicting politicians accused of war crimes, when in fact the blame and guilt attached to these crimes is wider reaching: "The old adage from Santayana that 'Those who don't learn from history are doomed to repeat it' is a lie" she meditates, "There is no history. Everything we are is eternally with us. Our question is therefore: What can save us from our crazy insistence on spreading the blight in ever widening circles?"

On closer examination *The Addiction* can be interpreted not only as an attempt to answer this question, but also as a rejection of the view that there is anything inevitable about this 'blight.' Conklin comes to realize this as she fights against accepting her fate as a bloodsucker and thus against the presupposition that we are all destined to commit acts of evil. These two points of view are embodied in the film by the characters of Peina and Conklin's professor. Peina is a vampire who after fasting for forty years, has been able to control his habit by exercising will and self-discipline. He feeds off Conklin, but she manages to escape and rid herself of the influence he has over her. The professor delivers the following class on Protestant theology:

> One aspect of determinism is manifested in the fact that the unsaved don't recognize the sin in their lives. They're unconscious of it. They don't suffer the pangs of conscience, because they don't recognize evil exists. This is because they are all predestined to hell and therefore never brought to the light of Metanoia or conversion, which is a work of grace only in a believer's life. So in considering the salvatory aspect of facing guilt, suffering is a good thing. We should all hope to feel guilty to feel pain to seek pardon and ultimately freedom. Guilt is a sign that God is working out your destiny, and it's a foolish person who refuses to acknowledge this.

The temptation must be resisted to read this as the film's ideological standpoint. In fact, the exact opposite is the case. On hearing this talk, Conklin vomits blood and later says that her professor and those of his ilk, "are all liars. Let 'em rot with cancer, we'll see what they have to say about free will." She decides to pit "the violence of my will against theirs" by refusing to submit to her vampiric condition. *The Addiction* ultimately does not endorse a theology of positive suffering and guilt: even if vampires might stand for evil in general, Conklin's battle nevertheless indicates there is something that can be done about this situation. This is underlined by Conklin's transfiguration in the film's final sequence.

After one more orgy of blood-drinking, she collapses on the street and is rushed to hospital. From her hospital bed, she looks up at a crucifix on the wall and asks the nurse to open the blinds, allowing a bright white light to come into the ward. As Conklin's face is bathed in light, a female vampire enters the room and makes a desperate last-minute attempt to reverse Conklin's transfiguration by closing the blinds: "We're not evil because of the evil we do, but we do evil because we are evil" she says, "What options do such people have? It's not like we had any options." But there *is* an option, there is an alternative. Conklin confesses to a priest: "God, forgive me." She is administered the last rites and dies. A woman identical to Conklin walks away from her grave and a headstone on which is written, "I am the resurrection and the life" (John 11:25). Some might feel this to be an ambiguous ending, but I would interpret it as Conklin's rebirth and redemption: the "Amen" in voice-over indicates that her new life has already begun. This is how I would also interpret the film's final voice-over spoken by the 'new' Conklin: "To face what we are in the end, we stand before the light and our true nature is revealed. Self-revelation is annihilation of self." In this case the annihilation of Conklin as vampire before she is reborn and, if you like, cleansed. Ferrara has said that Conklin finds redemption at the end because, "she wants it. She wants to believe. She knows it. She's not a stranger to Christ."[13]

The Funeral (1996) was Ferrara's last collaboration with Nicholas St. John to date. Since then he has directed three more feature films along with a rock video and a five-minute segment for the compilation film *Subway Stories* (1997) entitled *Love On the A Train*. The promo music video "California" (1996) is another example of the Ferrara motif of vengeance. It features rock singer Mylène Farmer in the double role of a rich woman who recognizes her doppelgänger in an L.A. prostitute. When the hooker is murdered by her Hispanic pimp, the high-society woman slips into her role and takes revenge. *Love On the A Train* is a story of romantic deception, and this theme is picked up by 1997s *The Blackout*. After an alcohol and drug addicted Hollywood movie star takes an overdose and blacks out, we see him eighteen months later obviously 'clean' and living with a woman haunted by fantasies that he might have murdered his former girlfriend. Parallels to *Ms. 45*, *Bad Lieutenant* and *The Addiction* are clear in the way, "a descent into violence" is seen to be, "as much a process of self-discovery as dissolution."[14]

New Rose Hotel (1998) is based on a story by Cyberpunk novelist William Gibson. It depicts an apocalyptic world in the near future which is controlled by powerful companies - the border between business and crime has long been blurred. Ferrara's most recent film *R Xmas* (2001) set in 1993, is a gangster/kidnapping film that concentrates on the pressure one family has to endure until they are eventually pushed closer together. The central character is a variation on the Frank White character from

King of New York. Although an 'honest' drug dealer who is kind to his family and helps out the community, he is nevertheless oblivious to the fact that his so-called decent lifestyle does immense damage to the lives of others.

Finally, two new Ferrara projects have been announced. Franchise Pictures are to produce *Coup d'Etat*, written and directed by Ferrara: the story of a parallel universe in which independent filmmakers literally wage battle against the studios in a war-torn Hollywood. Also slated for production is the prequel to *King of New York* entitled *The Last Crew* which according to the director will explore the 'King's' background, his youth, and how he ended up in jail for the first time. According to Ferrara, in relation to his future projects and direction, "We're ready, we're rocking, we just want to keep the show on the road. Whatever it takes, we're not hung up on our, quote-unquote, 'cult reputation'."[15]

4.   Conclusion

Many critics have tried to grapple with the nature of the Abel Ferrara phenomenon. He has been called an anarchist and Catholic, to quote the subtitle of Danese's book, as well as "an artist of extravagance, of transgression, of outrage."[16] He has also been seen as an advocate of a form of critical mysticism, determined to reintegrate those subversive elements of Catholicism that have been suppressed in traditional Catholic iconography and faith.[17] Ultimately, any attempt to understand Ferrara's work without taking his spiritual and religious concerns into consideration is unproductive. When asked in an interview whether he uses his films in order to come to grips with questions of redemption, Ferrara replied:

> Of course. It's not my films, it's my life. A film is not a 90-minute thing. A film is everything that I am. We keep coming back to the point of, 'Who are we? Where do we come from? What's our future?' We do plenty of dealing with the now. But I don't know how you can fucking live and not question where you're from.[18]

Ferrara's search for redemption should also be seen in the context of embattled American Catholics who seek to confront the weight of a predominantly Protestant, if not downright Calvinist and Fundamentalist mind-set. Such religious conformity can be witnessed not only in churches across the country, but also in cinema and televangelism's fire and brimstone sermons with their promise of instant salvation (for a price). At the end of the 80s and throughout the 90s, a series of American films were released such as *Angel Heart* (1987) and 1995s *Se7en* [*sic*] which dealt with the origins of evil in its development of the disturbing and inescapable (often Calvinist) notion of sin and predestination: Calvinist in the sense that those singled out for punishment were constructed to more than deserve the fate awaiting them. This preordained damnation theology was in turn radically challenged by *Bad Lieutenant* and *The Addiction* with their claims to universal salvation. In the end, Ferrara's characters don't have an easy go of it. There is no instant salvation. According to Gavin Smith, in *The Blackout*: "the protagonist is once again submerged in self-consuming excess until reduced to a state of abjection, everything stripped away to prepare for decisive self-confrontation: it's the quintessential Ferrara experience."[19] Indeed it is.

Notes

1. International Abel Ferrara Internet Library, 2002, www.
2. In addition, The Ferrara Internet Library gives March 2001 presumably as the date of publication for a study by Brad Stevens entitled *The Moral Vision*, but the book won't appear until the end of the year. Book-length studies have also been written by Canova, Danese, Herrgott, and Pezzota.
3. While admitting that, "Ferrara's work splits into two halves: everything before *King of New York* and everything since", Johnstone goes on to structure his study around six "distinct sections: The Urban Victim Trilogy (*The Driller Killer, Ms. 45, Fear City*), The TV Years (*Miami Vice, Crime Story, The Gladiator*), The Territorial Trilogy (*China Girl, Cat Chaser, King of New York*), The Redemption Trilogy (*Bad Lieutenant, Snake Eyes, The Addiction*), High Budget Re-Make Disaster (*Body Snatchers*) and what could be called The Damnation Duo (*The Funeral, The Blackout*)." Some of the subsequent chapters have different headings the neatest of which is The Redemption Trilogy: "The Gospel According to St. John," i.e. Nicholas St. John (chapter 7). It is to the credit of Ferrara's art that the multifaceted nature of his films allows for all possible divisions and classifications. Johnstone, 1999, 2 and 4.
4. Kiefer and Stiglegger, 2000, 17.
5. St. John "has never written for any other director" and now "lives in New York State" where "he teaches Catholic catechism for a living, writing the screenplays around this full-time commitment." Johnstone, vii.
6. Johnstone discusses the question of whether *The Nine Lives Of A Wet Pussy* from 1975/76 can really be considered a genuine part of the

Ferrara oeuvre while Kiefer and Stiglegger mention that the film is known more as a 'legend' and reproduce three stills from it. Johnstone, 7-8; Kiefer and Stiglegger, 18.

7. There are three books in his room: *Thus Spoke Zarathustra* by Nietzsche, Darwin's *The Origin of Species*, and *Crime and Punishment* by Dostoevsky. In addition, Pazza writes down every new attack in a journal with the words FEAR CITY in red on the cover. Pazza therefore predates the philosophically inclined serial killer John Doe from *Se7en* by a good decade. Doe not only structures his murders around the Medieval seven deadly sins, but he also keeps a journal in which he maniacally writes down his thoughts. Similar to Pazza, Doe candidly verbalizes the justifications for his deeds though to the two detectives working the case, not in voice-over. A further parallel is the way both Pazza and Doe abhor what they believe are the filth and scum they see on every urban street and take it upon themselves to 'clean things up.'

8. The lieutenant telling Rossi he is a 'hero' at the end of *Fear City* could equally be regarded as an act of forgiveness and remission of sins.

9. Johnstone, 116.

10. Smith, 1997, 9.

11. Schuppach, 2000, 166.

12. Kiefer/Stiglegger, 9.

13. Smith, 9.

14. Newman, 1998, 41.

15. Cited in Johnstone, 1999, 36.

16. Lyons, 1994, 22.

17. A summary of Danese in Kiefer/Stiglegger, 2000, 13.

18. Smith, 9.

19. Smith, 6.

References

Canova, Gianni (1997), *Abel Ferrara*. Rome: n.p.

Danese, Silvio (1998), *Abel Ferrara - l'anarchico e il cattolico*. Genoa: n.p.

Ferrara, A. (director). (2001), *R Xmas*. [film]. Franchise Pictures. USA. and France

—— (1998), *New Rose Hotel*. [film]. Entertainment and Edward R. Pressman. USA.

— (1997), *The Blackout*. [film]. Edward R. Pressman, MDP Worldwide, CIPA and Les Films Number One. USA. and France.

— (1997), *Subway Stories: Love On The A Train*. [television]. HBO. USA.

— (1996), *The Funeral*. [film]. C&P Productions, MDP Worldwide and October Films. USA.

— (1994), *The Addiction*. [film]. Fast Films Inc. USA.

— (1993), *Body Snatcher: The Invasion Continues*. Warner Bros. USA.

— (1993), *Snake Eyes* [a.k.a. *Dangerous Game*]. [film]. Maverick Picture Company. USA.

— (1992), *Bad Lieutenant*. [film]. Distribution Ltd. and Edward R. Pressman. USA.

— (1990), *King of New York*. [film]. Reteitalia SPA and Scena International. USA.

— (1988), *Cat Chaser*. [film]. Vestron Pictures. USA.

— (1987), *China Girl*. [film]. Vestron Pictures, Street Lite, Great American Films Limited Partnership. USA.

— (1986), *The Gladiator*. [film]. Walker Brothers and New World Company. USA.

— (1984), *Fear City*. [film]. Zupnik-Curtis Enterprises. USA

— (1981), *Ms. 45*. [film]. Navaron Films. USA.

— (1979), *Driller Killer*. [film]. Navaron Productions. USA.

— (1975), *Nine Lives of a Wet Pussy*. [film]. Navaron Films. USA.

Fincher, D. (director). (1995) *Se7en* [*sic*]. [film]. New Line Cinema. USA.

Herrgott, Elizabeth (1999), *Le destin d'Abel ou an outburst of love*. Paris: n.p.

International Abel Ferrara Internet Library (1 August, 2002), http://www.miscellanea.de/film/Abel_Ferrara.

Johnstone, Nick (1999), *Abel Ferrara: The King of New York*. London/New York/Paris/Sydney: Omnibus Press.

Kiefer, Bernd, and Marcus Stiglegger (2000), 'Abel Ferrara und die Suche nach Erlösung', in: Kiefer/Stiglegger (eds.), *Die bizarre Schönheit der Verdammten: Die Filme von Abel Ferrara*. Marburg: Schüren. 9-40.

Lyons, Donald (1994), *Independent Visions*. New York: n.p.

Newman, Kim (1998), rev. of *The Blackout, Sight and Sound*, 8.3: 40-41.

Parker A. (director). (1987), *Angel Heart* [film]. Carolco Entertainment, Union and Winkast. USA, Canada and UK.

Pezzota, Alberto (1998), *Abel Ferrara*. Il Castro Cinema: n.p.

Schuppach, Sandra (2000), 'Der Kopf und der Körper: Christopher Walken und Harvey Keitel als 'acteurs fétiches',' in: Kiefer/Stiglegger (eds.). *Die bizarre Schönheit der Verdammten*. 159-69.

Smith, Gavin (1997), 'Dealing with the now,' *Sight and Sound*, 7.4: 6-9.

Stevens, Brad (forthcoming), *The Moral Vision*.n.p.

Notes on Contributors

Meg Barker
Meg lectures in Psychology and Media and Cultural Studies at University College, Worcester. She researches in the areas of identity and the representation of gender and evil. She would like to thank Sue Chesters, Vicky Bateman and Darren Oldridge for their invaluable help, and the Pagans and Goths who gave so much time and support.

William A. Cook
William resumed the Professor's role in 2000 after 13 years as Vice President for Academic Affairs at the University of La Verne in southern California. He spent the 2000-2001 academic year in Europe researching the Cathars and giving lectures at the University of Gloucestershire in Cheltenham, England. He currently teaches Advanced Writing for English Majors, American Literature, and Literature and Mythology for the English Department. His last book is *A Time to Know*, London: Routledge, 2000.

Paul Davies
Paul is an English language instructor at the University of Passau, Germany, where he teaches courses on essay writing, translation, and English-language film. He holds an MA from the University of Manitoba and a Ph.D from Queen's University. His research interests include spirituality and religion in film, women filmmakers, and the aesthetics of TV series.

Loren Glass
Loren is Assistant Professor of American Literature and Cultural Studies at Towson University, USA.

Madelaine Hron
Madelaine is a doctoral student at the University of Michigan - her Ph.D. is on *The Translation of Pain in Immigrant Texts*. Though her work focuses mostly Czech and French literature, she is also concerned with human rights issues, representations of violence, and trauma and healing in literature and art.

Rebecca Knuth
Rebecca is an Associate Professor in the Library and Information Science Program at the University of Hawaii. She has recently written, *Libricide: The Regime-Sponsored Destruction of Books and Libraries in the Twentieth Century*. New York: Praeger (forthcoming)

Earl F. Martin
Earl is a Professor of Law at Texas Wesleyan University School of Law in Fort Worth, Texas. Professor Martin holds a J.D. from the University of Kentucky and an LL.M. from The Yale Law School.

Diana Medlicott
Diana is Reader in Crime and Penology at Buckinghamshire Chilterns University College, UK. Her main research areas are penology, restorative justice, and place identity.

Darren Oldridge
Darren lectures in History, Media and Cultural Studies at University College Worcester. He has published extensively on early modern history, most recently as the editor of *The Witchcraft Reader* London: Routledge 2002. Darren would like to thank Dr. Meg Barker for her invaluable help with his contribution to this book

Fiona Peters
Fiona is completing a PhD on Patricia Highsmith in the School of English at the University of Gloucestershire. Her MA is in Critical Theory from the University of Sussex and she was Principal Lecturer in Critical Theory at the University of North London. She has taught Philosophy and Literature at the Universities of Sussex and Middlesex. At present she teaches Critical Theory and Film Studies at the University of the West of England, Bristol.

Michael F. Strmiska.
Michael holds a Ph.D. in Religious Studies from Boston University. He lecturers in World Religion at Miyazaki International College, Miyazaki, Japan.

Terrie Waddell
Terrie is a lecturer in Media Studies at La Trobe University, Victoria, Australia. Her research interests and publications focus on myth, ritual, carnival, grotesqueries, advertising, and the representation of women in media. Originally trained as an actor, she has worked in film, television, theatre and radio.

The University of Crisis

Edited by David Seth Preston

Amsterdam/New York, NY 2002. XV,226 pp.
(At the Interface/Probing the Boundaries 1)

ISBN: 90-420-1570-5   € 45,-/US $ 45.-

This book began as a collection of papers presented at a conference entitled 'The Future Business of Higher Education' held at Oxford University. The contributions range from those who grapple with the question of what a University should do, through those concerned with making Higher Education more efficient, to some who were already planning for some technologically inevitable virtual future. These disparate leanings led to inevitable conflict and a challenge in editing into book form. In compiling and editing the chapters the editor has tried to preserve some of the diversity of opinion presented at Oxford. By doing so it is apparent that some individual contributors would find unacceptable much of what others in the book have to say. The traditionalists clash with the modernizers, the Left with the Right, Public with Private and the theorists with the practitioners. It is this very divergence of philosophical opinion as to the future of Higher Education that makes this book such an enjoyable and stimulating read.

USA/Canada: One Rockefeller Plaza, Ste. 1420, New York, NY 10020,
Tel. (212) 265-6360, *Call toll-free* (U.S.only) 1-800-225-3998,
Fax (212) 265-6402
All Other Countries: Tijnmuiden 7, 1046 AK Amsterdam, The Netherlands.
Tel. ++ 31 (0)20 6114821, Fax++ 31 (0)20 4472979
orders-queries@rodopi.nl   **www.rodopi.nl**

Understanding Evil:
An Interdisciplinary Approach.

Edited by Margaret Sönser Breen

Amsterdam/New York, NY 2003. XIII, 222 pp.
(ATI/PTB 2)

ISBN: 90-420-0935-7   € 45,-/US $ 45.-

Written across the disciplines of law, literature, philosophy, and theology,
Understanding Evil: An Interdisciplinary Approach represents wide-ranging
approaches to and understandings of "evil" and "wickedness."
Consisting of three sections – *"Grappling with Evil"*
"Justice, Responsibility, and War" and *"Blame, Murder, and Retributivism,"*
- all the essays are inter-disciplinary and multi-disciplinary in focus. Common
themes emerge around the dominant narrative movements of grieving, loss,
powerlessness, and retribution that have shaped so many political and cultural
issues around the world since the fall of 2001.   At the same time, the
interdisciplinary nature of this collection, together with the divergent views of
its chapters, reminds one that, in the end, an inquiry into "evil" and
"wickedness" is at its best when it promotes intelligence and compassion,
creativity and cooperation.
The thirteen essays are originally presented at and then developed in light of
dialogues held at the Third Global Conference on Perspectives on Evil and
Human Wickedness, held in March 2002 in Prague

USA/Canada: One Rockefeller Plaza, Ste. 1420, New York, NY 10020,
Tel. (212) 265-6360, Call toll-free (U.S. only) 1-800-225-3998,
Fax (212) 265-6402
All other countries: Tijnmuiden 7, 1046 AK Amsterdam, The Netherlands.
Tel. ++ 31 (0)20 611 48 21, Fax ++ 31 (0)20 447 29 79
Orders-queries@rodopi.nl   www.rodopi.nl

Suffering, Death, and Identity

Edited by Robert N. Fisher, Daniel T. Primozic, Peter A. Day, and
Joel A. Thompson

Amsterdam/New York, NY 2002. XI,210 pp.
(Value Inquiry Book Series 135)

ISBN: 90-420-1173-4   € 40,-/US $ 40.-

This book explores many of the issues that arise when we consider persons
who are in pain, who are suffering, and who are nearing the end of life.
Suffering provokes us into a journey toward discovering who we are and
forces us to rethink many of the views we hold about ourselves.

USA/Canada: One Rockefeller Plaza, Ste. 1420, New York, NY 10020,
Tel. (212) 265-6360, Call toll-free (U.S. only) 1-800-225-3998,
Fax (212) 265-6402
All other countries: Tijnmuiden 7, 1046 AK Amsterdam, The Netherlands.
Tel. ++ 31 (0)20 611 48 21, Fax ++ 31 (0)20 447 29 79
Orders-queries@rodopi.nl   www.rodopi.nl

Legal and Political Philosophy
Social, Political, & Legal Philosophy, Volume 1

Edited by Enrique Villanueva

Amsterdam/New York, NY 2002. XII,481 pp.
(Rodopi Philosophical Studies 5)

ISBN: 90-420-1103-3   € 100,-/US $ 100.-

LEGAL AND POLITICAL PHILOSOPHY, edited by Enrique Villanueva, is the first volume in the series Social, Political, and Legal Philosophy, published by Rodopi also under his editorship. It contains six original essays by leading political philosophers and philosophers of law (Waldron, Coleman, Postema, Shapiro, Sayre-McCord, and Kraus), along with critical papers on those essays, and replies. This is cutting edge work that elicits sharp responses already as it is published, with the debate joined as the authors reply.

SOCIAL, POLITICAL AND LEGAL PHILOSOPHY is a new book series, edited by Enrique Villanueva, and published by Rodopi Publishers as part of Rodopi Philosophical Studies. The series will publish collections of new essays on topics in social or political or legal philosophy. New volumes will be published approximately every year or every other year.

USA/Canada: One Rockefeller Plaza, Ste. 1420, New York, NY 10020,
Tel. (212) 265-6360, Call toll-free (U.S. only) 1-800-225-3998,
Fax (212) 265-6402
All other countries: Tijnmuiden 7, 1046 AK Amsterdam, The Netherlands.
Tel. ++ 31 (0)20 611 48 21, Fax ++ 31 (0)20 447 29 79
Orders-queries@rodopi.nl   www.rodopi.nl

Touching Philosophy, Sounding Religion, Placing Education

Steven Schroeder

Amsterdam/New York, NY 2002. VI,122 pp.
(Value Inquiry Book Series 136)

ISBN: 90-420-1163-7   € 27,-/US $ 27.-

This book redefines religious studies as a field in which a plurality of disciplines interact. A social science when understood as a body of knowledge, religion is also marked by discovery, appreciation, orientation, and application—an interplay of the arts and sciences. Teaching religious studies involves the question of the occupation of territories and disentangling occupation from violence.

USA/Canada: One Rockefeller Plaza, Ste. 1420, New York, NY 10020,
Tel. (212) 265-6360, Call toll-free (U.S. only) 1-800-225-3998,
Fax (212) 265-6402
All other countries: Tijnmuiden 7, 1046 AK Amsterdam, The Netherlands.
Tel. ++ 31 (0)20 611 48 21, Fax ++ 31 (0)20 447 29 79
Orders-queries@rodopi.nl   www.rodopi.nl

Feminism/Femininity in Chinese Literature.

Edited by Peng-hsiang Chen and Whitney Crothers Dilley.

Amsterdam/New York, NY 2002. X,219 pp. (Critical Studies 18)

ISBN: 90-420-0727-3   € 55,-/US-$ 55.-
ISBN: 90-420-0717-6   € 25,-/US-$ 25.-

The present volume of Critical Studies is a collection of selected essays on the topic of feminism and femininity in Chinese literature. Although feminism has been a hot topic in Chinese literary circles in recent years, this remarkable collection represents one of the first of its kind to be published in English. The essays have been written by well-known scholars and feminists including Kang-I Sun Chang of Yale University, and Li Ziyun, a writer and feminist in Shanghai, China. The essays are inter- and multi-disciplinary, covering several historical periods in poetry and fiction (from the Ming-Qing periods to the twentieth century). In particular, the development of women's writing in the New Period (post-1976) is examined in depth. The articles thus offer the reader a composite and broad perspective of feminism and the treatment of the female in Chinese literature. As this remarkable new collection attests, the voices of women in China have begun calling out loudly, in ways that challenge prevalent views about the Chinese female persona.

USA/Canada: One Rockefeller Plaza, Ste. 1420, New York, NY 10020,
Tel. (212) 265-6360, Call toll-free (U.S. only) 1-800-225-3998,
Fax (212) 265-6402
All other countries: Tijnmuiden 7, 1046 AK Amsterdam, The Netherlands.
Tel. ++ 31 (0)20 611 48 21, Fax ++ 31 (0)20 447 29 79
Orders-queries@rodopi.nl   **www.rodopi.nl**

In Words and Deeds
The Spectacle of Incest in English Renaissance Tragedy.

ZENÓN LUIS-MARTÍNEZ

Amsterdam/New York, NY 2002. VIII,296 pp. (Costerus NS 145)
ISBN: 90-420-0844-X   € 55,-/US $ 55.-

Departing from earlier studies which regarded incest as a literary topos or dramatic metaphor foregrounding political, social, or legal issues, *In Words and Deeds: The Spectacle of Incest in English Renaissance Tragedy* argues that the presence of incest on the Renaissance stage is a strategy for the enactment of the spectator's tragic experience. Incest is explored neither as a sin nor as a crime, but as an "unspeakable" experience filtered through dramatic words and deeds. The incitement of desire, visual pleasure, and unconscious fantasy, as well as traumatic rejection, pain, and horror, are all aspects of this paradoxical and uncanny experience. Aristotelian theory of tragedy, Freudian and Lacanian psychoanalysis, and Michel Foucault's notions of the deployment of sexuality and alliance, concur in the analysis of plays where incest is a central or a secondary motif – Ford's *'Tis Pity She's a Whore*, Beaumont and Fletcher's *Cupid's Revenge*, Webster's *The Duchess of Malfi* – and others where incest is an effect of language and *mise-en-scène* – Sackville and Norton's *Gorboduc*, Shakespeare's *King Lear*. The variety of topics and the combination of critical perspectives makes *In Words and Deeds* an attractive book for students and teachers of Renaissance drama, as well as for those with a special interest in psychoanalytic and other new theoretical approaches to the literary text.

USA/Canada: One Rockefeller Plaza, Ste. 1420, New York, NY 10020,
Tel. (212) 265-6360, Call toll-free (U.S. only) 1-800-225-3998,
Fax (212) 265-6402
All other countries: Tijnmuiden 7, 1046 AK Amsterdam, The Netherlands.
Tel. ++ 31 (0)20 611 48 21, Fax ++ 31 (0)20 447 29 79
Orders-queries@rodopi.nl   www.rodopi.nl

Representing the Real

Ruth Ronen

Amsterdam/New York, NY 2002. VI,218 pp.
(Psychoanalysis and Culture 11)

ISBN: 90-420-0973-X   € 40,-/US $ 40.-

This study offers a new perspective on the object represented by art, specifically by art that successfully creates in its recipient a sense of "the real", a sense of approximating the true nature of the represented object that lies outside the work of art.

The object that cannot be accessed through a concept, a meaning or a sign, the thing-in-itself, is generally rejected by philosophy as being outside the realm of its concerns. This rejection is surveyed in a number of philosophical discussions, from Kant to Hilary Putnam. Turning to the psychoanalytic object, an object which cannot be exhausted in terms of its external existence or conceptual status or meaning (the object is always suppressed, partly known, inaccessible), introduces another notion of the object. The Real is suggested as that which can neither be contained in language nor reduced to a linguistic referent. This solution does not lead away from philosophical interests but rather exposes this dilemma engendered by the object of representation as fundamentally philosophical.

Cases of artistic realism discussed range from perspective painting to abstract art, from tragedies to the literary representation of minds.

USA/Canada: One Rockefeller Plaza, Ste. 1420, New York, NY 10020,
Tel. (212) 265-6360, Call toll-free (U.S. only) 1-800-225-3998,
Fax (212) 265-6402
All other countries: Tijnmuiden 7, 1046 AK Amsterdam, The Netherlands.
Tel. ++ 31 (0)20 611 48 21, Fax ++ 31 (0)20 447 29 79
Orders-queries@rodopi.nl   www.rodopi.nl

Dimensions of Health and Health Promotion

Edited by Lennart Nordenfelt and Per-Erik Liss

Amsterdam/New York, NY 2003. XV,225 pp.
(Value Inquiry Book Series 138)

ISBN: 90-420-0924-1   € 45,-/US $ 45.-

This book contains scholarly contributions to several current debates in the philosophy of medicine and health care regarding the nature of health and health promotion, concepts and measurements of mental illness, phenomenological conceptions of health and illness, allocation of health care resources, criteria for proper medical science, the clinical meeting, and ethical constraints in such a meeting.

With one exception, the authors in this book are or have been teachers or graduate students at the interdisciplinary Department of Health and Society (Tema H) at Linköping University, Sweden. While all the texts have a philosophical focus, many other disciplines have influenced the choice of specific perspectives. The university backgrounds of the authors range from medicine, psychology, sociology, and religion to philosophy. What binds the authors together is their deep interest in the theory of medicine and in the pursuit of a philosophy of humanistic medicine and health care.

USA/Canada: One Rockefeller Plaza, Ste. 1420, New York, NY 10020,
Tel. (212) 265-6360, Call toll-free (U.S. only) 1-800-225-3998,
Fax (212) 265-6402
All other countries: Tijnmuiden 7, 1046 AK Amsterdam, The Netherlands.
Tel. ++ 31 (0)20 611 48 21, Fax ++ 31 (0)20 4 47 29 79
Orders-queries@rodopi.nl   www.rodopi.nl

Singularity and Other Possibilities
Panenmentalist Novelties

Amihud Gilead

Amsterdam/New York, NY 2003. X,245 pp.
(Value Inquiry Book Series 139)

ISBN: 90-420-0934-9   € 50,-/US $ 50.-

This book elaborates the author's original metaphysics, panenmentalism, focusing on novel aspects of the singularity of any person. Among these aspects, integrated in a systematic view, are: love and singularity; private, intersubjective, and public accessibility; multiple personality; freedom of will; akrasia; a way out of the empiricist-rationalist conundrum; the possibility of God; and some major moral questions.

USA/Canada: One Rockefeller Plaza, Ste. 1420, New York, NY 10020,
Tel. (212) 265-6360, Call toll-free (U.S. only) 1-800-225-3998,
Fax (212) 265-6402
All other countries: Tijnmuiden 7, 1046 AK Amsterdam, The Netherlands.
Tel. ++ 31 (0)20 611 48 21, Fax ++ 31 (0)20 447 29 79
Orders-queries@rodopi.nl   www.rodopi.nl

Nursing Ethics in Modern China
Conflicting Values and Competing Role Requirements

Samantha Mei-che Pang

Amsterdam/New York, NY 2003. XIII,265 pp.
(Value Inquiry Book Series 140)

ISBN: 90-420-0944-6   € 52,-/US $ 52.-

This book follows two lines of inquiry in understanding nursing ethics in the historical-cultural context of modern China. Firstly, it scrutinizes the prescribed set of moral virtues for nurses in fulfilling their role requirements during different periods of nursing development over the past century. Based on empirical studies, the book, secondly, explores the nurses' evaluations of their ethical responsibilities in current practice. It carefully examines the particular viewpoints of nurses in their ethical appraisal of nursing practice and patient care situations. Drawing upon traditional ethical outlooks, international norms, and the experiences of nurses as they face difficult care situations, this book concludes with recommendations for improving the quality of nursing in contemporary China.

USA/Canada: One Rockefeller Plaza, Ste. 1420, New York, NY 10020,
Tel. (212) 265-6360, Call toll-free (U.S. only) 1-800-225-3998,
Fax (212) 265-6402
All other countries: Tijnmuiden 7, 1046 AK Amsterdam, The Netherlands.
Tel. ++ 31 (0)20 611 48 21, Fax ++ 31 (0)20 447 29 79
Orders-queries@rodopi.nl   www.rodopi.nl